The Numb Foot Book

The Numb Foot Book:

How to Treat and Prevent Peripheral Neuropathy

Volume 4 in the Numb Toes Series

by
**Alexander McLellan, ND and
Mark Spitz, DPM**

MedPress
Halifax, Nova Scotia

Published by
MedPress, PO Box 81, Halifax, Nova Scotia, Canada, B3J 2L4
www.medpress.com

ISBN: 978-0-9781820-5-2

This text is printed on acid-free paper.

Printed in the United States of America.

10 9 8 7 6 5 4 3 2

To my neuropathy patients, who have inspired me with their resilience to adversity, commitment to healing, and willingness during adverse times to reach out and help others in pain.

\- Alexander McLellan, ND

Dedicated to Sharon—my wife and best friend, and my beautiful daughter Leah Rose.

\- Marc Spitz, DPM

Contents

Contents

Contents

The Numb Foot Book

Figures and Tables

Foreword

A decade of living with at least three types of neuropathy (carpal tunnel syndrome, diabetic neuropathy and lumbar radiculopathy) finds me remembering so many moments of overwhelming pain-filled fear and despair. Happily I can also say there are a lot of really wonderful memories of liberating symptom relief and the pure joy of pursuing a new vocation as a neuropathy support group leader, researcher, writer, activist and advocate. But I am just one of hundreds of laypersons working to educate and support other PNers (i.e., those with peripheral neuropathy) in the support group network of the Northern California Chapter of The Neuropathy Association, and others across the U.S. and world. However much we've learned and shared with others, our work is far from over. We still encounter newcomers who haven't a clue as to what has hit them, and there are far too many "old timers" who've been suffering mostly alone for 20, 30, maybe even 40 years with their mysterious conditions. Whether "youngish" or "oldish," far too many have had little significant treatment help, patient education or emotional support from their medical providers, families, or fellow PNers, much less the general public. After all, neuropathy still remains one of the most common diseases most have never heard of and all too few of us understand even a small portion of its multifarious realities at any meaningful level.

And yet progress really is being made; many of us are getting effective help for our weird sensations, fears and confusion. Times really are changing, thanks to the hard work of many in the medical and neuropathy patient advocacy communities. The appearance now of this very marvelous volume, "The Numb Toes Book" by Alexander McClellan, ND, and Marc Spitz, DPM, is the latest cause to celebrate these ever changing and more hopeful times.

Their unique expertise and sensibilities from the medical fields of naturopathy and podiatry bring very relevant perspectives we need to know and appreciate in our quest for comprehensive understanding. Their accumulated data and wisdom brings us exciting next levels of observations and synthesized models of new developments in research we need to know about. Their use of very identifiable personal stories from across the neuropathy experience spectrum reassures us that we really aren't alone and there really is cause for hope. These are very significant accomplishments for a small, but really quite excellent book that adds much needed clarity to the neuropathy literature.

I can't imagine what it must have been like trying to contend with neuropathy *BJS*, that is, *Before John Senneff,* whose marvelous research and very readable ground-breaking three books, the "Numb Toes…" series began in 1999 to illuminate our darkness. Some of us were blessed to be involved in support groups across America associated with The Neuropathy Association (TNA) and were reading Senneff's books as they became available through TNA and traditional market resources. We were profoundly grateful for his growing knowledge and positive vision that life really is possible with neuropathy. Many diabetic (and other) neuropathy patients were astounded to learn that when we acted upon his insights about nutrients, exercise and various treatment options, we really did reduce and sometimes reverse our symptoms.

Later on we began to surf the net for more information, desperately trying to make greater sense of our specific situations. While most of us were usually dismissed as having "idiopathic" neuropathy, some of us were coming to understand that good diagnosticians could define us more precisely and there were more effective treatments, if only we and our doctors could learn more. We were amazed to see the reams and reams of available information on the Internet or the long list of text books found on Amazon, etc. Especially when our doctors kept telling us, "We just don't know much about neuropathy... it's just a part of getting older...your nerves are dead...we don't know why...we really don't have much to help you." And indeed, most didn't, and all too often still don't. But some of us were learning there was knowledge and there was help, as we took heed of and built upon Senneff's pioneering work.

Our reality is that neuropathy is an incredibly complex multi-faceted condition that defies all our efforts to make it simple and controllable. Acknowledging and affirming that reality is just one of the great benefits of the book at hand. Grasping some of the many different aspects of neuropathy – the causes, signs and symptoms, treatment options, and still largely unknowable prognoses, we come to understand there probably can be no one single book that puts it all together in clear, non-technical language, while addressing all our concerns and needs.

My hunch is that it would take a few thousand pages in several volumes. For instance, there are reportedly about 100 different types of neuropathy, as represented in TNA's 1999 publication, *A Guide to the Peripheral Neuropathies*. But there are also some 200 distinct causes many of which were elucidated in the 2007 guidebook for patients and families by Norman Latov, MD,

PhD, *Peripheral Neuropathy When the Numbness, Weakness and Pain Won't Stop.* Furthermore, there are ever growing numbers of evolving theories of just why X, Y and Z causes are damaging our nerves, leaving some of us with severe disabilities, but others doing quite well with minimal difficulties. And we certainly wonder why some specific treatments – prescribed or over-the-counter, really work marvelously well for some of our biochemistries but are total failures for others. There are no simple answers for who, what, why, where and how of our neuropathies.

It is not enough to be told, "Well, neuropathy is not a simple single disease, it's more like a gargantuan configuration of disorders with seemingly endless variables impacting different parts of our bodies, literally from head to toe, with our information processing brains affecting us in different and often unpredictable ways." One of the extraordinary beauties of this book is that so many questions, with their very complex implications, are expertly but intelligibly addressed. One comes away with many "Aha!" moments in suddenly realizing that some frustrating knot has unraveled before our eyes. We gradually become empowered to get our arms around our generally common and distinctly personal realities with neuropathy. Embracing arms <u>and</u> comprehending arms, for they are both essential for our restoration to better health. Only then can our overpowering sense of dread and hopelessness begin to subside.

Somehow we'll be able to see and say: "OK, maybe all that does make sense. Maybe we need to pay attention to our weight and pre-diabetic or actual diabetes condition because we really don't want to have those horrible complications. Maybe we'll quit being passive patients and start really learning about our conditions and entering into a partnership relationship with our doctors. Maybe it's time to abandon our childish demands for a magic pill for a cure and give the topicals and other alternative treatments a chance. Maybe we'll give up our couch potato life styles and get up to walk, do tai chi, and other exercises, trusting we can learn to not fall again as we strengthen our weak muscles and know sensation is being restored. Although we may be scared of needles, maybe acupuncture really could relieve our pain. Even if we'd much prefer steak and potatoes, maybe there really is something to eating wisely with lean protein, lots of colorful fruits and vegetables, whole grain fiber and the right kinds of fats. Biochemistry may well be far beyond us, but maybe those antioxidants and other supplements really can help us."

And then, just maybe, we'll stop thinking and acting in terms of "maybes" and get on with taking concrete, positive actions as suggested by Dr. McClellan and Dr. Spitz. We'll likely find we feel and function a whole lot better if we learn and embrace their vital and essential lessons.

The neuropathy community will be truly blessed by and grateful for the labor of love presented in *The Numb Toes Book*, thanks to Dr. McClellan and Dr. Spitz. And thanks to MedPress Publications Inc. and Origin BioMed, Inc. for bringing it to us for the sake of our good health and restored lives.

Martha Chandley, MA
Neuropathy Support Group Leader, Educator and Advocate
West Sacramento, California
April 2008

The Numb Foot Book

Chapter 1

Introduction

Peripheral neuropathy affects 20 million Americans, yet most people have never heard of this condition. In fact, peripheral neuropathy continues to be under-diagnosed, under-treated, and under-researched—a frustrating situation for sufferers, their families and doctors.

One of the frustrating aspects of peripheral neuropathy is the fact that peripheral neuropathy sufferers usually do not exhibit any outward signs of the disease, such as redness or swelling. Thus it is often difficult for outsiders to relate to the extreme discomfort brought about by peripheral neuropathy. Doctors, friends, and family cannot see your pain. It is, therefore, easy for others (including health insurance companies) to minimize the sometimes life-altering effects of the disorder. At the same time, the costs to society of peripheral neuropathy are staggering. Billions of health care dollars are spent every year managing this condition. The cost in terms of loss of mobility and lost productivity is even higher and more difficult to quantify. Even greater are the human costs such as loss of quality of life, difficulty maintaining valuable social and family relationships, and coping with the depression that often accompanies long-term pain and suffering.

Although testing for peripheral neuropathy has become more sophisticated and accurate, many questions and problems still confront the patient, even after the diagnosis is made. Two of the more commonly asked questions are: "What caused my condition?" and "What is my outlook?" That is, will my condition improve, stay the same or worsen?

Current pharmaceutical treatment options may not adequately relieve the symptoms of peripheral neuropathy or may lead to worrying side effects. This also contributes to a great deal of concern, worry and stress for neuropathy sufferers and their loved ones.

If you have peripheral neuropathy, or someone close to you has it, you have probably already experienced the frustrations which can accompany this disorder. For many there is the initial frustration of getting an accurate diagnosis. Because symptoms can vary from mild tingling to excruciating pain, and may include unusual sensations or problems with balance, patients may go for months without proper treatment and care. Others may be diagnosed but lack an understanding of the condition, be unsure of its alternative treatments, be unaware of simple self-care solutions or just hunger for information in general.

This book was created primarily as a guide for the person with peripheral neuropathy. Our main goal is quite simply to help you understand your condition and its treatments. You will find information in straight-forward language about how the nervous system works and how damage to nerves leads to neuropathy. It is our intention to help you understand how the diagnosis of peripheral neuropathy is made and which medical tests may help your doctor to make the diagnosis. There is also an extensive focus on treatment options, including the advantages and disadvantages of various drug treatments, physical treatments (infrared therapy, laser, TENS, etc.) and alternative treatments (massage therapy, nutritional supplements, acupuncture, etc.).

You will also hear from many peripheral neuropathy sufferers as they share their personal experiences and treatments that worked for them. For example, in an entire chapter devoted to diabetic peripheral neuropathy, you will find out how nutritional supplements and diet helped a person who had diabetes for more than 35 years. A chapter devoted to walking and balance problems includes, in the patients' own words, many personal experiences of how neuropathy affects daily life. And, in the chapter dedicated to nutritional supplements for neuropathy, there is a case report detailing how an early-stage neuropathy was reversed.

Additionally, there's in-depth information on nutrients and vitamins commonly used to treat the various symptoms of PN.

We hope this book sheds light on peripheral neuropathy in many ways. By understanding peripheral neuropathy better, we hope you are better able to discuss your symptoms and options for treatment with your health care practitioners. Although there is no magic cure right now for peripheral neuropathy, we encourage optimism and action. At best, you may be able to reverse your symptoms; at least, you may be able to slow or stop the disorder's progression. Finally, we hope with this book to raise awareness of peripheral neuropathy, and to double the efforts of the peripheral neuropathy associations that work hard to support the community of neuropathy sufferers.

Chapter 2

Explaining Peripheral Neuropathy

What Is Peripheral Neuropathy?

Peripheral neuropathy refers to a series of medical conditions affecting the nerves outside the brain and spinal cord. The brain and spinal cord comprise the central nervous system which is the "computer" of the nervous system—coordinating and processing information. The peripheral nervous system connects the brain and spinal cord to skin, muscles, tendons and internal organs. Damage to the nerves of the peripheral nervous system causes the condition of peripheral neuropathy.

You Have Some Nerve! What They Look Like and How They Work

The main component of the peripheral nervous system is called the neuron. A neuron is a nerve cell that sends and receives elec-

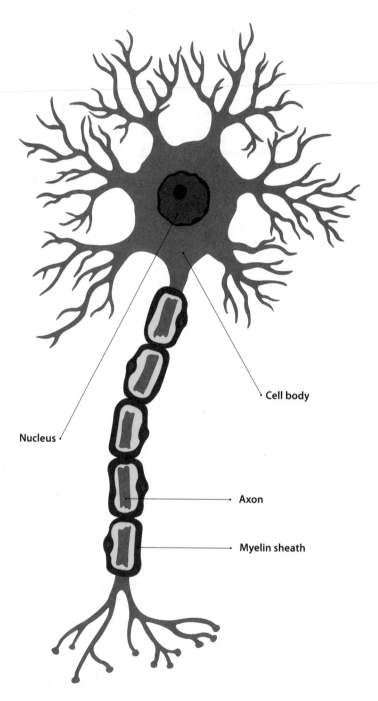

Cell body

Nucleus

Axon

Myelin sheath

Fig. 1: The Neuron

trical signals. It carries information that allows different parts of the body to communicate with each other.

Each neuron is made up of a cell body with a long tail called the axon. The cell body receives and processes nerve signals and sends these signals through the axon to the end of the neuron, called the axon terminal. The axon terminal then releases chemicals called neurotransmitters, which allow the nerve signal to "jump" to the next neuron. The transmission of nerve impulses from one nerve to the next is called an electrical synapse.

Axons are similar in structure to common electrical wires. Like electrical wires, axons have a protective covering called the myelin sheath. Myelin protects the nerve and insulates the axon so it can conduct electrical impulses faster and more efficiently. Axons travel together in bundles called nerve trunks.

Three Types of Nerves of the Peripheral Nervous System

The peripheral nervous system is made up of three different types of nerves. Damage to two types of nerves, sensory and motor nerves, causes most of peripheral neuropathy symptoms. Sensory nerves carry information from the brain and spinal cord to sense receptors located in the skin and other areas in the body. These nerves allow us to feel pain, hot and cold sensations, vibrations and touch. They also communicate with the brain so we have the ability to sense the position, location and movement of our body parts. This ability is called proprioception.

Many people with peripheral neuropathy develop loss of sensation, which often results in the more common symptoms of peripheral neuropathy including, pain, tingling, numbness and burning. With the loss of proprioception we lose the ability to feel where our feet are positioned relative to the ground. This causes loss of balance with severe walking difficulties.

Motor nerves carry information away from the brain and spinal cord to the muscles and are responsible for voluntary movement. Damage to the motor nerves usually occurs in later stages of peripheral neuropathy process. Motor nerve disturbances can cause muscle weakness, walking difficulty, muscle cramps, a feeling of "heaviness of the feet and legs" and a condition called drop foot. People with drop foot cannot raise their foot at the ankle and tend to "drag" the affected foot or in some cases both feet. This makes walking extremely challenging.

Damage to the sensory and motor nerves primarily affects the lower extremities—legs, feet and toes. It is less common for people to develop neuropathies that simultaneously affect both the feet and hands. Persons with diabetes are more prone to developing neuropathies of the upper and lower extremities. One common neuropathy that affects the wrist and hand is carpal tunnel syndrome.

The final nerve type of the peripheral nervous system is called the autonomic nerve. Autonomic nerves control the involuntary muscles of the internal organs and glands. They are responsible for the proper functioning of our lungs, heart, digestion, glands and sexual function. Damage to the autonomic nerves can cause cardiovascular, bladder, bowel and sexual dysfunction.

Mono-Poly-Diabetic Neuropathies—In English Please!

Some people experiencing symptoms of peripheral neuropathy undergo a nerve study ordered by their physician, neurologist or podiatrist. A common positive finding of a nerve study might read something like this, "This study is abnormal indicating moderate lower extremity polyneuropathy characterized by evidence of axon loss." Experiencing peripheral neuropathy can be frightening enough, yet the terminology associated with the condition can certainly add to the anxiety.

Polyneuropathy

Polyneuropathy accounts for the greatest number of peripheral neuropathy conditions. Poly is derived from Greek and means "many." Polyneuropathies occur when one or more nerve types (sensory, motor and autonomic), are simultaneously damaged. They are usually symmetric—meaning that both sides are affected. It should be noted that even though most polyneuropathies are symmetrical, it is common to experience greater symptoms on one side of the body. A person with peripheral neuropathy may experience burning and tingling in both feet, yet one foot may have stronger and more uncomfortable sensations than the other. When just the motor and sensory nerve fibers are affected, the condition is called "sensorimotor neuropathy."

Persons with diabetes are particularly prone to developing polyneuropathies. A person with diabetic polyneuropathy may have numbness and loss of sensation in the feet (sensory nerve damage), muscle weakness (motor nerve damage) and sexual dysfunction (autonomic nerve damage).

Mononeuropathy

Mononeuropathy is damage to a single nerve or nerve group, with injury being the most common cause. Nerve injury is often caused by prolonged and repeated pressure on a nerve. Nerves that run close to bony prominences are most vulnerable to injury. Besides injury, there are many other causes of mononeuropathies. These include:

- Certain chemotherapy drugs and radiation therapy for cancer treatment

- Exposure to toxic substances such as solvents, lead, arsenic and mercury

- Some prescription medications, such as statin drugs to control high cholesterol levels and some antibiotics used to treat infections

- Infections such as Lyme disease and AIDS

- Exposure to extreme temperature changes—frostbite, for example, may cause permanent nerve damage

The most common mononeuropathy is carpal tunnel syndrome. This condition occurs from repetitive, strenuous activities and injury to the wrist. Repetitive motion over an extended period of time such as computer users who hold their wrists in a fixed position for many hours a day, are prone to developing carpal tunnel syndrome.

Carpal tunnel syndrome occurs when the median nerve, which runs from the forearm into the hand, is damaged by excessive pressure. The median nerve actually runs through a natural "tunnel" formed by ligaments at the base of the hand. Continual pressure or injury on this structure causes the tunnel opening to narrow, thus pinching the nerve. This can result in numbness, burning, tingling, "pins and needles" sensation, weakness and pain.

Tarsal tunnel syndrome is the foot's counter part to carpal tunnel syndrome. It is due to injury to the tarsal nerve of the ankle. Bell's Palsy is a mononeuropathy affecting a cranial nerve causing weakness or paralysis to the facial muscles. Other forms of mononeuropathy include sciatica, radial and ulnar damage to nerves in the upper extremity and peroneal nerve palsy affecting a major nerve around the knee. Peroneal nerve injury may lead to drop foot, a condition causing severe walking problems.

What Causes Peripheral Neuropathy?

As discussed, peripheral neuropathy is due to damage to the nerve cells and nerve fibers. Nerves can be damaged in two ways: The cover of the nerve, the myelin sheath, can be stripped away or the "tail" of the nerve, the axon, can be destroyed. Peripheral neuropathy is usually an acquired condition but in some cases it may be inherited.

Diabetic Neuropathies

Diabetes is the most common cause of peripheral neuropathy. It can lead to serious complications and will be addressed in a later chapter as well. It is estimated that approximately 50 percent of all persons with diabetes develop some form of peripheral neuropathy. Several factors have been implicated as to why persons with diabetes develop neuropathies in far greater proportion than the general population. Hyperglycemia—high blood glucose (sugar) levels causes chemical changes which results in damage to the nerve cells. In effect, the nerve just like electrical wire "short-circuits." The damaged nerves lose their ability to conduct nerve impulse properly. Elevated blood glucose levels also damage the blood vessels that carry oxygen and nutrients to the nerves. Researchers have also postulated that autoimmune factors may cause inflammation in nerves. This means that a person's immune system may attack its own nerve cells. Studies have also shown that persons with diabetes with high blood sugar levels may inhibit the production of nitric oxide. Nitric oxide dilates or opens blood vessels, thus increasing circulation. People with diabetes appear to have lower levels of nitric oxide which reduces circulation, causing damage to the peripheral nerves.

Neuropathies Caused by Chemotherapy

The development of peripheral neuropathy following chemotherapy treatment is a fairly common occurrence. Chemotherapy agents that aggressively "attack" cancer cells often have a neurotoxic effect, damaging the nerve cells as well. The extent of nerve damage depends on the cumulative dose and the type of

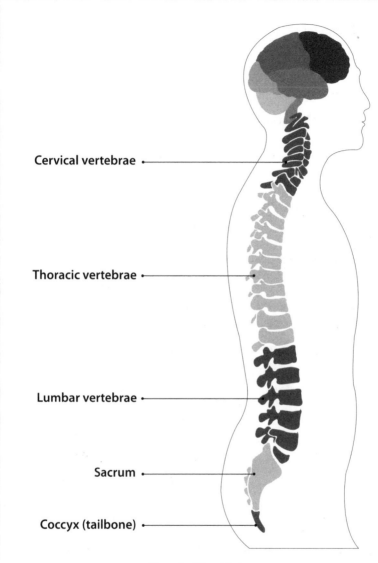

Fig. 2: The Spine

- Cervical vertebrae
- Thoracic vertebrae
- Lumbar vertebrae
- Sacrum
- Coccyx (tailbone)

drugs used. Symptoms include pain, burning, numbness, tingling and muscle weakness. Recovery from these symptoms is often incomplete. Taxol®, a drug frequently used in the treatment of breast, ovarian, lung, head and neck cancers, has been known to cause chemotherapy-induced neuropathy. Other chemotherapy drugs that can cause nerve damage include Cisplatin and Vincristine.

Neuropathy Caused by Spinal Problems

The spinal cord runs through and is protected by the spinal column. The spinal column consists of interlocking bony segments called vertebrae. The vertebrae extend from the brain stem to the tail bone.

Ideally the spinal cord, made of many millions of nerve fibers, should run through the spinal column without interruption. Spinal stenosis is a condition whereby the spinal column is narrowed. Stenosis can be caused by injury, arthritis or scoliosis. A narrowed spinal column places excessive pressure on the spinal cord nerves. The nerves of the upper spine, in the region of the cervical vertebrae, affect the upper extremities—arm, wrist, hand and fingers. The nerves in the lumbar and sacral regions affect the lower extremities—the large sciatic nerve, legs, feet and toes. Neuropathy symptoms of pain, tingling, numbness and burning are manifested in the area of spinal damage. Spinal stenosis in the cervical part of the spine might cause numbness of the fingers, which would mimic symptoms of carpal tunnel syndrome. Stenosis of the lower spine, in the lumbar-sacral area, might cause pain and numbness in the feet and toes.

Neuropathy Caused by Excessive Alcohol Intake

Prolonged and excessive use of alcohol will invariably have a toxic effect on nerve tissue. Studies have shown that the incidence of alcoholics who develop peripheral neuropathy ranges from 25 to 50 percent. Nutritional deficiencies often associated with alcohol abuse can exacerbate neuropathy symptoms.

Neuropathies caused by Toxins and Drugs

As noted previously, exposure to certain toxins such as arsenic, lead, mercury, thallium, chemical solvents and nitrous oxide, can cause nerve damage. Some insecticides may also cause peripheral neuropathy symptoms. Certain anticonvulsant, antiviral and antibiotic drugs may result in pain, burning, tingling and numbness. Drugs implicated in causing nerve damage include AZT, an antiviral medication used in the treatment of HIV infection. Gentamicin ciprofloxacin and levofloxacin are antibiotics used to treat a variety of infections. Nitrofurantoin and metronidazole (Flagyl®) are other classes of antibiotics used in the treatment of polynephritis, peritonitis and other infections. Phenytoin (Dilantin®) and carbamazepine (Tegretol®) are considered anticonvulsant drugs used to treat seizures and other disorders. All of the above mentioned drugs may be toxic to the peripheral nerves.

Neuropathies Caused by Nutritional Imbalance

Deficiencies of vitamins B12(cobalamin), B1(thiamine), B6 (pyridoxine) or vitamin E can cause peripheral neuropathy symptoms. Vitamin B12 plays an important role in neurologic function. Although the exact prevalence is not known, studies have shown that up to 15 percent of the adult population may have vitamin B12 deficiency. It is far more common in adults over 65 years and the condition can be exacerbated by gastric antacid medication.

It should also be noted that overuse of some vitamins may actually cause peripheral neuropathy. This includes taking megadoses of B6 and B12. Caution should also be used when taking higher doses of vitamin E as well, since this is a fat-soluble vitamin and can accumulate in the body's tissue. A later chapter in this book will discuss nutritional therapy and recommended dosages.

Neuropathies Caused by Infection

It is estimated that nearly one-third of people with HIV/AIDS experience peripheral neuropathy. Nerve damage can be caused by the medication, the actual virus or a combination of both. Common drugs that have nerve-damaging potential include Epivir®, Retrovir® (also known as AZT), Ziagen®, Droxia®, Hivid®, Videx® and Zerit®.

Hepatitis, a viral infection primarily affecting the liver, may cause nerve damage. Lyme disease, which is a bacterial infection transmitted to humans by the bite of a black-legged tick, can also cause neuropathy.

Neuropathies Caused by Autoimmune Diseases

As noted previously in this chapter, an autoimmune disease is a condition in which the immune system destroys or attacks its own bodily tissues. The following is a list of autoimmune diseases that can cause peripheral neuropathy:

- Rheumatoid arthritis: A chronic disease marked by stiffness, inflammation of the joints and loss of mobility.

- Systemic lupus erythematosus: A chronic autoimmune disorder that can affect the skin, joints, kidneys and other organs.

- Guillian-Barre syndrome: A rare autoimmune disorder that attacks and destroys peripheral nerves. It can be triggered by trauma, pregnancy, infection or a vaccination. Chronic inflammatory demyelinating polyneuropathy(CIDP) is thought to be another form of this syndrome. CIDP is a condition whereby the protective cover of the nerve, the myelin sheath, is destroyed by the immune system.

Neuropathies Caused by Cancer

Different types of cancers can have varying effects on nerves. Multiple myeloma is a type of cancer that affects the plasma cells in the bone marrow. It can cause destruction to the axon part of the nerve cell. Certain blood cancers—chronic lymphocytic leukemia and lymphoma—can also cause peripheral nerve damage. Small-cell lung cancer can have an adverse effect on sensory nerves. As noted earlier in this chapter, neuropathy frequently develops as a consequence of chemotherapy treatment.

Neuropathy Caused by Hereditary Conditions: Charcot-Marie-Tooth Disease (CMT)

Charcot-Marie-Tooth disease is the most commonly inherited neurological disorder that affects approximately 150,000 people in the U.S. Damage to the peripheral nerves is caused by gene mutation. The condition is slowly progressive, causing numbness, tingling and burning. CMT primarily affects the motor nerves—those responsible for movement of the body. Damage to the motor nerves results in weakness of the foot and lower leg muscles and upper extremities as well. CMT often causes severe balance problems, high arches, hammertoes, foot bone deformities, loss of hand function and drop foot deformity.

Neuropathy Caused by Injury

Injury or excessive pressure on a particular nerve can result in nerve damage causing peripheral neuropathy symptoms. The most common neuropathy in this category is carpal tunnel syndrome. This syndrome is due to excessive pressure on the median nerve that supplies the wrist and hand. Symptoms include pain, weakness, tingling and numbness in the wrist and hand.

Sciatica is a condition due to nerve injury or excessive pressure on the sciatic nerve, a large nerve originating in the lower back and then branching into the lower leg. It is often caused by pressure on the sciatic nerve resulting from a herniated disc (referred to commonly as a slipped or ruptured disc). Spinal stenosis or narrowing of the spinal column can also cause injury to the sciatic nerve.

Symptoms of sciatica include:

- Pain in the buttocks area or leg that is worse when sitting

- Burning, tingling and numbness down the leg

- Weakness and difficulty moving the leg or foot

- A "shooting" pain radiating down the leg to the level below the knee

- Low back pain

Injury to the peroneal nerve—a major nerve supplying the legs, feet and toes can cause significant neuropathy symptoms. Common causes of peroneal nerve injury include damage to the knee, fracture of a leg bone, habitual leg crossing, and injury to the lower leg during surgery. Injury to the peroneal nerve can result in numbness, burning and tingling on the top of the foot. Other symptoms include weakness of the ankles or drop foot deformity.

Other Causes of Peripheral Neuropathy

There are many other medical conditions that have been linked to peripheral neuropathy. Amyloidosis is a group of diseases in which the body accumulates abnormal proteins. This protein called amyloid, can be deposited in nerve tissue causing neuropathy symptoms.

Other conditions include:

- Sarcoidosis: An inflammatory process causing small "lumps" to accumulate in body tissue.

- Sjögren's syndrome: An autoimmune disease in which extra antibodies can "attack" various tissues in the body.

- Kidney disease: Specifically chronic renal failure.

- Hypothyroidism: An underactive thyroid can lead to degeneration of the nerve cell.

Idiopathic Neuropathies

Neuropathies in which no specific cause can be identified are called idiopathic neuropathies. Often such neuropathies occur in people over 60-years-old. Studies have shown that a third of all neuropathies can be classified as idiopathic neuropathies.

Chapter 3

Symptoms and Diagnosis

Symptoms of Peripheral Neuropathy

The medical literature lists the symptoms of peripheral neuropathy as pain, numbness, burning, tingling and muscle weakness. This one sentence does not come close to describing the discomfort, misery and altered life style brought about by neuropathy. It is extremely difficult to accurately describe peripheral neuropathy symptoms. How do you articulate to someone that your feet are numb and painful at the same time? These two sensations seem like complete opposites, yet many peripheral neuropathy sufferers experience both.

Adding to this frustration is the fact that peripheral neuropathy is a "silent" disorder. This means that often there are no physical signs such as redness or swelling. Although there are sophisticated nerve tests (which will be discussed later in this chapter), the most important factor in diagnosing peripheral neuropathy is the person's own account of his or her condition.

Since a concise description is often so difficult, this presents a major challenge for the physician and family members.

The Foot Pain Center in Seal Beach, California, focuses on the diagnosis and treatment of peripheral neuropathy. The center sees hundreds of patients a year—most of whom have difficulty describing their peripheral neuropathy symptoms. To help the reader gain a better understanding of peripheral neuropathy symptoms, actual cases will be presented in which the patients describe their symptoms in their own words.

Case 1 "BW" 64-year-old female

"My feet feel numb yet they tingle and burn.

This all started about six years ago. At first I noticed a slight tingling at the ends of my toes. It didn't happen all the time, so I ignored it. Then I started noticing that is was happening almost every day. Over the next few years the sensation traveled to the soles of my feet. Now my feet feel as if they are asleep—kind of a numb feeling—but they also burn and feel like pins and needles are sticking into my toes. I almost wish they were just plain numb because I can't take the burning and tingling. The feelings are not consistent and some days are worse than others."

Case 2 "GL" 48-year-old male

"My feet are completely numb —I can't feel a thing.

I am a person with diabetes and having been using insulin for the past twenty years. Soon after I was diagnosed with diabetes my feet and toes started to feel numb. By the time I was about 35-years-old I could hardly feel anything in my toes, feet or ankles. I used to go barefoot around the house. One day I stepped on a carpet tack and didn't even feel it. A few weeks later I noticed blood on my sock. When I looked at my right foot (referring to injured foot), I saw that it was infected. My family doctor sent me to wound care center. They told me at the wound center that if does not heal properly that I could loose my foot. I had treatments three days a week. It took about seven months and the infection finally healed up. I learned my lesson from that experience and I always wear slippers around the house now."

Case 3 "SL" 67-year-old female

"My feet are so hot they feel like they are burning up.

I have been told that I have peripheral neuropathy. My feet are not numb nor do they tingle. My feet always feet hot. I cannot even stand the bed covers to touch them. I can't wear closed shoes and I even wear sandals in the winter—people think that I am crazy for doing this. The burning gets even worse in warm weather in rooms that heated too high in temperature. To get relief I sometimes stick my feet in a bucket of ice water."

Note: A word of caution—extreme temperature changes especially in those with poor circulation or diabetes, should be avoided as this can lead to serious foot complications. Complications include, worsening of the condition, or the risk of infections and foot ulcerations.

Case 4 "AR" 71-year-old male

"The burning and tingling in my feet is much worse at night—sometimes it is so bad that I can't get to sleep.

The pain and tingling in my feet is 10 times worse at night. I feel some discomfort during the day but it nothing compared to what I feel in the evening. I dread going to bed because my feet are so much worse at night. When I lie still I get terrible burning and stinging in my feet. I try changing positions or getting up and walking around. Sometimes this helps a little but mostly the burning and prickly sensations start up again."

Case 5 "LW" 79-year-old male

"When I walk, I feel like I am walking on marbles or sandpaper or cardboard.

It is the strangest feeling. It feels like I have something in my sock—sometimes it feels like my sock is bunched up. I stop what I am doing and take off my shoes and inspect my socks. I never find anything in my shoe or sock. I have purchased many different kinds of shoes and socks made out of different materials. This odd feeling never goes away no matter what I wear on my feet."

Case 6 "TR" 44-year-old female

"I developed burning and tingling in my fingers and toes after my chemotherapy.

Two years ago I was diagnosed with breast cancer and underwent three months of chemotherapy. My oncologist used a combination of drugs to treat the cancer. He told me about the possible side effects including numbness in my feet and hands. About three weeks into the treatments, my fingers and toes started to feel tingly and prickly. I told my doctor about this and he said the uncomfortable feelings might go away in time. He prescribed a medicine called gabapentin. It made me feel very groggy and tired and I had to stop taking it. I have noticed some improvement but my fingers and toes still burn and tingle."

Case 7 "LS" 69-year-old male

"I feel like I am wearing socks or slippers even though my feet are completely bare.

I could swear I am wearing something on my feet. It feels like a tight band around my feet and ankles. I just want to peel it off—of course, when I look down, there is nothing to peel off."

Case 8 "AD" 57-year-old female

"My feet are so cold that they feel like ice cubes.

My feet are always cold. There is practically nothing I can do to warm them up. I have my husband feel my feet and he tells me that they do not feel cold to him. When I go to bed I put two or three covers over my feet and they still feel freezing. I also try wearing thick socks and even two layers of socks. This does not help either."

Note: As noted previously, it is important to avoid extreme temperature changes. One case at the Foot Pain Center involved a 65-year-old insulin dependant person with diabetes. He experienced both coldness and numbness. In an effort to warm up his feet, he placed a heating pack in the microwave oven and placed it on his left foot. Having almost complete loss of sensation, this patient developed third degree burns on the foot.

Case 9 "JP" 76-year-old male

"My feet feel heavy and my hands are so weak that I can hardly turn the knob to open the front door at my house.

I developed peripheral neuropathy from drinking too much alcohol in my younger years. My feet feel as if they have lead weights attached to them. Just walking around the block takes a major effort. I dread walking upstairs at home. I have lost strength in my hands and fingers. I can't open the lids on most jars anymore. I seem to always be dropping things like my keys."

Case 10 "CC" 68-year-old female

"I feel very unsteady when I walk. I lose my balance and have fallen quite a few times.

I definitely have numbness, tingling and burning in my feet. I can live with this discomfort. It's the unsteadiness and loss of balance that makes life so difficult. I always feel like I am going to fall. In fact I have fallen about four or five times. Luckily I have not broken any bones yet. I get scared when I have to go to the bathroom in the middle of night because I am always afraid of falling. It is much worse in the dark because I can't see my feet or sense where I am going. I walk very slowly and feel better when I can hold on to something."

The ten cases just presented should give the reader a clear idea of the many different ways in which peripheral neuropathy can affect an individual. I continually hear new and descriptive terms for neuropathy symptoms: "SL" states that he feels as if "electric shocks are shooting into my legs and feet" while "RW" compares the sensations on the bottom of his feet to "walking on hot coals." The list of descriptions is practically endless. In medical terms the description of symptoms by the patient is called subjective findings. To further substantiate and verify the diagnosis of peripheral neuropathy, further testing is necessary. These results are called objective findings and will now be addressed.

Diagnosing Peripheral Neuropathy

The Clinical Examination

Following obtaining a detailed history, the clinical examination is the next important step in determining if a person has peripheral neuropathy. The purpose of the examination is to determine if in fact the patient has peripheral neuropathy, the extent of the nerve damage, the cause, which nerves have been affected, the prognosis and a treatment plan.

> **Testing the presence or absence of vibratory sensation:** Diminished or absent vibratory sensation indicate underlying neuropathy. For this test, a tuning fork is activated then placed on different locations on the foot.
>
> **Testing reflexes using a reflex hammer:** Deep tendon reflexes are responses to muscle stimulation. The areas most commonly tested are the knee, ankle, forearm, biceps and triceps. A crisp, reactive movement of the stimulated body part is the normal reaction. A weak or absent response (hyporeflexia), indicates peripheral neuropathy, muscle weakness (myopathy), or spondylosis (degeneration of the spine). Conversely, an overactive response (hyperreflexia) also indicates nerve disease such as spinal cord damage or severe brain trauma.

Testing proprioception: Proprioception is the body's ability to sense position and movement of the limbs. People with normal proprioceptive sense can navigate in the dark because they know where there feet are relative to the ground and their environment.

People with diminished proprioception cannot feel where they are and consequently have severe balance problems. Diminished proprioception is a cardinal sign for peripheral neuropathy.

Testing is performed as follows:

1. A person will close his or her eyes

2. The examiner grasps the sides of the great toe

3. The examiner then randomly moves the toe in an upward or downward position

4. The person being tested should be able to correctly identify the movement and direction of the toe being tested

Semmes-Weinstein Pressure Sensation Test

One of the most important clinical tests to help determine the presence of peripheral neuropathy is the Semmes-Weinstein Monofilament Test. A thin plastic wire (about the thickness and appearance of fishing line) is pressed against certain designated areas on the toes and feet.

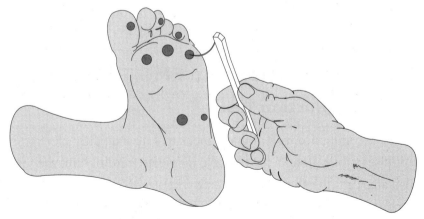

Fig. 3: Semmes-Weinstein Pressure Sensation Test

The examiner then asks the person being tested if he or she can feel the pressure of the wire. If the person cannot feel the touch of the wire that person is classified as having loss of protective sensation—a sign of peripheral neuropathy.

Muscle Testing

Peripheral neuropathy can affect both the nerves necessary for feeling, the sensory nerves and the nerves that allow movement of body parts, motor nerves. As a general rule, peripheral neuropathy initially affects the sensory nerves and as the condition progresses the motor nerves become involved as well. Damage to the motor nerves results in muscle weakness and loss of muscle bulk (muscle atrophy). An important part of the diagnostic examination is determining muscle strength. Muscle strength is graded from zero to five. Zero indicates complete absence of muscle strength. Five is normal muscle strength. The other numbers indicates varying degrees of muscle strength. Common areas tested are the wrist, fingers, thighs, knees, calves, ankles and toes.

Diagnostic Testing: Nerve Conduction and EMG Testing

Nerve Conduction Test

A nerve conduction velocity test measures how quickly electrical impulses move along a nerve. Like an electrocardiogram, the test also analyzes the shape of the nerve impulse. Healthy nerves will conduct an electrical impulse from the area being stimulated to a second recording site along the nerve or muscle innervated by the nerve. Motor nerves will also conduct impulses back to the spinal cord where they will bounce back and conduct down to the recording site. Normal time values are dependant on the age, sex, height and weight of the individual being tested. Delays in nerve conduction to the spinal cord as recorded by the nerve conduction testing device, indicates nerve damage. The test is performed as follows: Surface electrodes are placed over the nerve being tested and then stimulated with a small electric current for recording purposes. The velocity at which the nerve impulse is transmitted through the nerves is measured and recorded. Most nerve conduction is from one point on a nerve to another point or from one point on the nerve to the muscle. A healthy nerve will conduct signals with greater speed than a damaged nerve.

Nerve tests are extremely valuable in determining if the nerve is damaged and also the extent of the damage. Nerve damage is classified as follows: no damage, mild, moderate or severe. The standard testing protocol has been with needles or electrodes. Neurometrix® has developed a testing device called NC-stat® that uses a sensor pad instead of individual surface electrodes. It is highly accurate, easy to perform and the results are obtained immediately.

Electromyogram (EMG) Study

An electromyogram (EMG) measures the electrical activity of muscles at rest and also during movement (called contractions). An EMG helps diagnose damage to muscle tissue and nerves supplying the muscles. If there is damage to the nerves innervating a specific muscle, it will register on an EMG study. This is very helpful in the assessment of peripheral neuropathy. An EMG is also important in diagnosing other muscle disorders not caused by peripheral neuropathy, such as myasthenia gravis. The EMG test is performed by inserting a small sterilized needle into the muscle being tested. The presence or absence of muscle activity is recorded and reviewed by the physician.

Chapter 4

Diabetic Peripheral Neuropathy

Introduction

Diabetes is a disease in which the conversion of the food we eat into energy is altered. In a healthy individual, glucose molecules extracted from food enter the cells of the body so that the glucose can be used as energy or stored for the future as fat. This transfer of glucose from the bloodstream to the cells is facilitated by insulin, a hormone secreted by the pancreas. If you or someone you know has diabetes, it means that this process is altered in a way that results in increased levels of glucose remaining in the blood. There are two main ways in which this can occur. One possibility is that the pancreas may have been damaged by one's own immune system or toxic exposures, such that it can no longer produce adequate amounts of insulin. Without adequate insulin production, glucose cannot efficiently pass from the blood into the cells, and hence the level of glucose in the blood rises. This type of condition is known as type 1 or insulin-dependant diabetes. Another possibility is that the pancreas secretes adequate or even excess amounts of insulin, but the cells of the body have become less responsive to it. This is called type 2 diabetes or insulin-resistant diabetes. Either way, the result is blood glucose levels which can soar dangerously high and lead to severe diabetic complications or even death.

Before the discovery of insulin, type 1 diabetes was a fatal disease with no known methods of treatment or prevention. In the early 1920s two Canadians, Dr. Frederick Banting and Dr. Charles Best, discovered that a pancreatic extract had anti-diabetic action on dogs. They quickly focused on the purification and production of insulin, which was tested on the first human in 1922. While insulin does not cure diabetes, it has saved millions of lives by allowing for the long-term management of this condition. Nevertheless, research into the mechanisms of diabetes, its effective management, and the search for a cure continues. It is estimated that the cost to society in the United States alone surpasses $250 billion, including medical costs, disability and premature mortality (CDC National Diabetes Fact Sheet 2005). As most of us are aware, the rate of diabetes continues to rise. The World Health Organization predicts that diabetes will affect some 300 million people worldwide by the year 2025. And since 5.2 billion people worldwide are believed to be prediabetic or undiagnosed, these statistics are likely to swell. In North America, which is experiencing a unique demographic shift as the post-war baby boomers reach retirement, the rate of diabetes is predicted to double in the next 10 years. At the same time children in western societies are spending more and more time in front of computer, TV and video game screens and less time engaged in physical activity. This has resulted in pre-teens and teens experiencing the largest percentage increase in type 2 diabetes.

Why are Persons with Diabetes More Prone to Peripheral Neuropathy?

The most common cause of neuropathy in the developed world is diabetes. Depending on the source, it is estimated that 40 to 60 percent of all persons with diabetes have some form of neuropathy. This means that today there are likely over 20 million North Americans with diabetic neuropathy. Not all these people have been diagnosed with neuropathy, however, because they may not yet be experiencing symptoms or they may not have brought their symptoms to the attention of their physicians. Diabetic neuropathy is more common in people who have had diabetes for longer periods (seven years or more), have more problems managing their blood sugars, are over 40 years of age, are overweight or obese, have high cholesterol, or have high blood pressure.

There are a number of mechanisms that lead to tissue damage in persons with diabetes. One mechanism is similar to the "browning" or "carmelizing" effect we see when we cook with sugar in the kitchen. Chemically, sugars are binding to proteins and damaging these proteins irreversibly. In persons with diabetes, circulating sugar in the blood binds to proteins such as those found in blood vessels, reducing circulation to the nerve cells which impairs healthy nerve function and repair.

This phenomenon of protein damage by sugar molecules ("glycation") also damages other tissues as well, especially tissue found in the kidneys, connective tissue (joints/ligaments, etc.) and even cholesterol transport proteins (LDL). The reduced effectiveness of cholesterol clearance contributes to atherosclerosis in persons with diabetes.

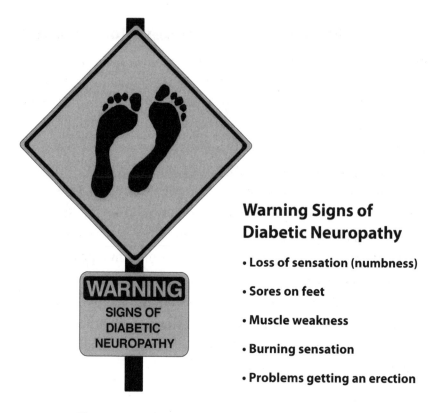

Fig. 4: Warning Signs of Diabetic Neuropathy

Another mechanism which leads to complications in persons with diabetes is the entry of excess glucose from the blood into tissues of the lens, nerves and kidneys. These tissues are poorly equipped to process this excess glucose, leading to the buildup of a byproduct of glucose called sorbitol. This excess sorbitol damages the cells, leading to cataracts in the lens, nerve damage and kidney damage. The enzyme which converts glucose to sorbitol in these tissues, aldose reductase, is one target of new natural and drug therapy for diabetic complications. Molecules that inhibit this enzyme hold promise for the management of these types of diabetic complications.

Incidentally, you may recognize that sorbitol is also marketed as a sweetener in many food and candy items. These types of sweeteners, including maltitol, mannitol, xylitol and lactitol, are also known as polyols. They are naturally in plant products, such as fruits and vegetables, and are safe for persons with diabetes to consume in moderate quantities (less than 10 grams per day). Sugar alcohols have a lower glycemic index than sucrose (table sugar) but are similar to sucrose in their sweetness. They also provide fewer calories (about 1/4 to 1/3 fewer calories) than regular sugar, thereby promoting healthy weight management. Sorbitol consumed in moderate amounts is metabolized by tissues of the body capable of breaking it down, such as the liver, so that it does not accumulate inside cells causing damage. However, sugar alcohols, like fructose in fruit and fruit juice, can have a laxative effect. Some persons with diabetes have also observed that their blood sugars rise if sugar alcohols are eaten in excess amounts.

Why is it Important to Control Blood Sugar?

Much research has confirmed that blood sugar control is one of the keys to preventing diabetic complications. Even those debilitated with all the complications of diabetes can see benefits from achieving better blood sugar management. Yet, in general, control of blood sugar in persons with diabetes is often less than optimal. Studies show only 25 percent of people with type 2 diabetes can achieve good (not even excellent) control with oral hypoglycemic medications. And once medications are begun, lifestyle, diet, nutrients, and herbs which can all contribute to better control are often ignored. In addition, without these other types of interventions, medications often lose their effectiveness even when the dose required to manage blood sugars reaches the maximum allowable.

One of the best ways to measure the success of a blood sugar management program is a blood test called glycosylated hemoglobin (HbA1c). HbA1c measures the effects of glucose on proteins found in the red blood cells. Recall that glucose can damage proteins in the process known as glycation, which is similar to the carmelization described earlier. By measuring the amount of sugar coating the red blood cells, one can get an idea of what the average blood sugar levels are. Since red blood cells live for an average of three months, HbA1c levels reflect average blood glucose levels during a three month time period. Therefore, HbA1c levels help assess how well an individual is controlling glucose levels on average. Since all of us, persons with diabetes and persons without diabetes, have glucose in our blood, all humans have some level of glycosylated hemoglobin. An HbA1c level below six percent is considered healthy and represents a good target for persons with diabetes to achieve. Even a level below seven percent has been shown to decrease the odds of diabetic complications. Conversely, higher levels of HbA1c have been associated with erectile dysfunction, eye disease (retinopathy), neurological disease such as peripheral neuropathy, coronary heart disease and overall increased risk of death.

It should be noted however that good blood sugar control is not only about a good average blood sugar. Averages sometimes hide daily ups and downs, and persons with diabetes must be encouraged to monitor their blood sugars and strive to keep them within the optimal range.

Why is it Important to Halt the Progression or Reverse Diabetic Neuropathy?

Peripheral neuropathy accounts for more hospitalizations than all other complications of diabetes, with a reported annual cost of more than $37 billion in the US. The individual cost in terms of loss of mobility, lost productivity and higher mortality rates is even higher and more difficult to quantify. The symptoms of neuropathy, which can range from mild tingling to excruciating pain, can affect all aspects of life. Indeed, some patients are unable to work, walk, sleep or engage in normal social interactions; some can hardly wear shoes or clothes because any contact with the skin is experienced as an unbearable pain or burning (allodynia). Once it develops, diabetic peripheral neuropathy is often difficult to reverse, depending on the extent of the nerve damage. In addition, as with other types of neuropathy, it often fails to respond to standard analgesic interventions.

As diabetic neuropathy worsens, the risk of lower-extremity amputation greatly increases. The compromised circulation present in persons with diabetes can lead to thinning and dry skin, especially in the extremities. Persons with diabetes may also develop decreased muscle tone in the foot, and therefore increased pressure from bony surfaces. The compromised tissue in the extremities is more easily damaged by day-to-day wear and tear. With reduced sensation due to neuropathy, the person with diabetes may not be aware that any damage has even occurred. Since the immunity of persons with diabetes is also compromised, these minor wounds may lead to major infections, such as infection of the bone (osteomyelitis). This sequence of events leads to over 60,000 amputations per year in North America alone.

An Important Message about Pre-Diabetes, Insulin Resistance and Metabolic Syndrome

The symptoms of peripheral neuropathy are often the first symptoms of diabetes that many people experience. Numbness, tingling or pain prompts many people to set up the initial appointment with their doctor. This can often lead to the diagnosis of diabetes. However, studies have confirmed that many people with confirmed cases of peripheral neuropathy are actually not diabetic but "pre-diabetic." Unfortunately this diagnosis is often missed, since there is a great deal of literature which deals specifically with diabetes but less so with other, more subtle, blood sugar disorders. In North America, a diet high in refined carbohydrates, combined with an inactive lifestyle, is contributing to a growing number of people with insulin resistance, hypoglycemia, and metabolic syndrome (Syndrome X). This puts our population at risk for diabetic complications even before a diagnosis of diabetes is made. Many of these "pre-diabetic" patients, if they do report peripheral neuropathy symptoms, are likely labeled as having "idiopathic peripheral neuropathy," meaning that the cause is unknown.

Many people can develop the early stages of the complications of diabetes even before their measured blood glucose levels are consistently outside the standard normal fasting blood sugar test ranges. Therefore, from the perspective of both prevention and treatment of neuropathies, it is important to note that metabolic changes that precede the development of diabetes often occur many years before the disease actually manifests. In some cases, over a decade may pass between the time the first symptoms develop and the diagnosis of diabetes. Early recognition of early stage-blood sugar irregularities can therefore help prevent the development of full-blown diabetes and the ensuing complications. Unfortunately, as a society we have done a very poor job of diabetes prevention, as evidenced by the soaring rates of diabetes and pre-diabetic conditions.

Part of early recognition includes monitoring for fasting glucose levels and glycosylated hemoglobin levels in the high normal range. Even for those with excellent results on these tests, another test, called a glucose insulin tolerance test (GITT) may be indicated. In the GITT the person is asked to ingest a known quantity of glucose, following which their blood glucose levels and insulin levels are monitored to see how their body handles the glucose. If blood sugar levels remain high for an extended period, the person is deemed to have a form of pre-diabetes known as glucose intolerance. If insulin levels are higher than expected, they are deemed to have hyperinsulinemia. Both glucose intolerance and hyperinsulinemia are forms of pre-diabetes since they can eventually lead to insulin resistant diabetes (type 2).

Metabolic syndrome (or Syndrome X) refers to a cluster of signs and symptoms present in many people with problems metabolizing glucose. It is estimated that at least 25 percent and perhaps as many as 50 percent of North Americans currently have this metabolic issue, which is also a precursor to diabetes. In metabolic syndrome, excess insulin is released in response to a meal containing carbohydrates. This excess insulin release is associated with high blood pressure, high triglyceride levels, and low HDL ("good" cholesterol) levels, and is therefore a risk factor for cardiovascular disease. Predisposing factors include a family history of type 2 diabetes, diets high in carbohydrates and sedentary lifestyles. Truncal obesity, fatty liver, difficulty losing weight, and hypoglycemia often accompany this condition. The good news is that the treatments offered for the management of blood sugar in persons with diabetes will also benefit those with metabolic syndrome, often reversing the condition completely.

Hypoglycemia, or low blood sugar, is defined as blood glucose values that are less than 50 mg/dl (2.8 mmol/l). The diagnosis of hypoglycemia, however, is usually based on symptoms. This is because the blood sugar lows are transitory, and it is often difficult to get a blood sample taken at the moment people are experiencing symptoms. When there is a shortage of glucose supply to the brain the result can be confusion, irritability, and problems focusing and remembering. Extreme cases may even lead to fainting, convulsions and coma. Although many view hypoglycemia as the opposite of diabetes (or hyperglycemia), the two are often linked. For example, excess blood glucose after a meal can lead to excess insulin release (metabolic syndrome), and this excess insulin can drive blood sugar levels excessively low, leading to hypoglycemia. Hence, hypoglycemia should be taken seriously, as it also has been shown to be a precursor to diabetes.

Diabetes Diagnosis

The symptoms of diabetes are often general and many people therefore ignore them or confuse them with other illnesses. According to the National Institutes of Health (NIH), nearly 25 percent of diagnoses of diabetes are made during a routine physical examination. Excessive thirst and excessive urination are the symptoms most well known by the general public, however many persons with diabetes experience no symptoms at all. Nearly half of adults diagnosed with type 2 diabetes indicated that they had no symptoms of the disease at the time they were diagnosed. This is one reason that approximately half of all persons with diabetes remain undiagnosed. If you or someone you know is experiencing a vague collection of symptoms similar to those listed here, it's important to discuss them with a healthcare practitioner. The importance of screening for early signs and symptoms of diabetes, followed by regular physician visits including physical examinations for those diagnosed with diabetes, cannot be overemphasized.

Signs and Symptoms

Type 1 Diabetes

- Excess thirst and excess urination
- Excess hunger
- Weight loss despite a normal or increased dietary intake
- Fatigue
- Repeated fungal or other types of infections
- Blurred vision

Type 2 Diabetes

Usually comes on slowly

- Overweight or obese
- High blood pressure
- High cholesterol or triglycerides

- Family history of type 2 diabetes
- Diet high in refined carbohydrates, deficient in dietary fiber
- Lack of physical exercise
- Truncal obesity
- Skin tags
- Opportunistic infections

Hypoglycemia

- Hungry between meals or at night
- Symptoms are worse if a meal is missed and better after eating
- Insomnia, awakening with inability to return to sleep
- Indecision, foggy thinking if a meal is delayed or missed
- Poor memory
- Feeling overly emotional, angry or irritable
- Crave sweets, alcohol, caffeine, bread, pasta, potatoes, or other simple carbohydrates
- Headaches if a meal is delayed or missed
- Sleepy or drowsy after meals
- Fatigue relieved by eating
- Feel faint if meal is delayed
- Cold hands or feet
- Blurred vision or seeing spots
- Dizziness, giddiness, or lightheadedness

Preventing Diabetes

Lifestyle plays an important role not only in the management of diabetes but also in preventing the onset of diabetes. Based on studies of identical twins, it is believed that genetic factors alone account for as little as five to 15 percent of type 1 cases, and even less of type 2 cases. Dietary and environmental factors therefore play a much larger role in the development of diabetes than genetics. For example, the single strongest predictor of an individual's risk of developing type 2 diabetes is being overweight. And, conversely, physical exercise and dietary modifications have proven effective in delaying or preventing the disease. Knowing that diabetes is largely preventable, and that type 2 diabetes is often reversible, should serve as a motivator. By altering their lifestyle and following a program of nutritional supplementation, many people are able to achieve healthy blood sugars. In many cases of type 2 diabetes this can be achieved without reliance on pharmaceuticals. This may not be easy, but typically the earlier one begins the process, the better the results. People tend to underestimate the benefits of small incremental changes that, over time, can provide long-term health benefits. Try to avoid the trap of giving up if you are not meeting your own expectations 100 percent of the time!

Clinical Trial:
The Diabetes Prevention Program

This was the first study that showed that exercise and diet can effectively delay diabetes. A diverse American population of over 3,000 overweight people was put on a program of a healthy diet and more active lifestyle. These people were already experiencing glucose intolerance. Yet, lifestyle interventions reduced the rate of diabetes onset by a remarkable 58 percent. In fact, the results were so impressive that the trial was ended a year early, as it was deemed unethical to continue without allowing those participants in the trial who were not making the lifestyle changes (i.e., the control or placebo group) to get the benefit of knowing the trial results. Lifestyle intervention worked as well in men as in women and in all the ethnic groups tested. Remarkably, lifestyle intervention also worked well in people age 60 and older, a group in which 20 percent of people at any one time have been diagnosed with diabetes. In fact, their risk of diabetes was reduced by a whopping 71 percent. This type of result has been confirmed by other researchers and by clinical practice.

Lifestyle Factors Contributing to Insulin Resistance and Type 2 Diabetes

- High carbohydrate diet
- High saturated fat and trans fats diet
- High refined sugar and starch diet
- Diet high in foods that are high on the glycemic index
- Low protein consumption
- Diet very low in essential fatty acids
- Diet that is inadequate in fiber
- Diet deficient in micronutrients (such as chromium)
- Lack of physical activity
- Stress
- Smoking (nicotine consumption)
- Obesity and overweight

Table 1: Lifestyle Factors Contributing to Diabetes

Type 1 Prevention

In type 1 diabetes, also known as insulin-dependent diabetes mellitus (IDDM), the insulin-producing cells of the pancreas are damaged. The damage to the pancreas prevents the production of enough insulin to regulate blood sugar levels. Type 1 diabetes is called insulin dependent diabetes mellitus because it is necessary to supply insulin to the body on a regular basis. This is typically done by means of insulin injections.

In most cases, the first step in the development of type 1 diabetes is believed to be the development of an autoimmune reaction against the pancreatic beta cells. It has been found that this process of autoimmunity can start very early in life, often even in the first two years after birth. The immune response, it is believed, is triggered by an infection, toxin, or a food allergen. Once triggered, the overzealous immunity somehow mistakes the pancreas as a foreign invader. The ensuing "collateral damage" results in a slow destruction of the beta cells.

This type of diabetes is usually associated with an early onset (before age 30) and represents only about 10 percent of the North American persons with diabetes population.

Viral Infections

Infections may be one cause of type 1 diabetes mellitus. Researchers have noted that the onset of type 1 diabetes peaks at age 5 and 11, which may be related to an increase in viral exposures at school. Viruses which have been implicated as triggers for type 1 diabetes include Coxsackie viruses, mumps virus, echoviruses, rotaviruses and other enteroviruses. These viruses may damage the pancreas directly, leading to an autoimmune response against damaged pancreatic cells. It is also possible that the immune system, in fighting these viruses, "cross-reacts" and confuses healthy pancreatic cells with the invaders. A third possibility is that the virus damages the gastrointestinal tract, leading to an immune reaction to undigested food proteins, which then reacts against healthy beta cells. What is known is that 75 percent or more of type 1 persons with diabetes develop anti-pancreatic beta cell antibodies.

Although it is impossible for children to avoid viral infections, it is possible to ensure that their immune systems are as healthy as possible. Adequate vitamin and mineral intake, avoidance of refined and processed foods, and organic food consumption are all recommended. In addition, ensuring that children receive healthy "probiotic" bacterial supplements, especially during bouts of viral diarrhea or after antibiotic therapy, likely reduces the risk of "leaky gut" and immune system hyper-reactivity. Proper gut microflora are also believed to help prevent some of the gastrointestinal infections implicated in the development of diabetes.

Cow's Milk

Cow's milk ingested in infancy may contribute to the autoimmune response against the pancreas found in type 1 persons with diabetes. Researchers at McMaster University in Canada published a critical review of literature pertaining to cow's milk exposure and its relation to diabetes in Diabetes Care. They found that type 1 diabetes was correlated with early exposure to cow's milk and diminished breast-feeding. Their review concluded that the increased risk for diabetes may be 1.5 times higher for those children who were fed cow's milk before four months of age. Research published in The New England Journal of Medicine linked bovine serum albumin (BSA) to this autoimmune response. In one of the most convincing trials, called the "Trial to Reduce Diabetes in the Genetically at Risk" (TRIGR), researchers manufactured two indistinguishable formulas and instructed parents to use them after weaning. One group received a formula containing cow's milk protein; the other received formula in which the protein was broken down. Nearly five years later antibodies to the pancreas were found in 22 percent of the children receiving cow's milk, compared to only 13 percent of the group receiving the predigested milk proteins. The presence of these antibodies correlates nearly 100 percent to the development of type 1 diabetes before puberty.

Researchers at the Hospital for Sick Children, Toronto, published two interesting studies that provided evidence of similarities between type 1 diabetes, multiple sclerosis and an immune reaction to cows' milk. The research, published in 2001 in *The Journal of Immunology*, noted that although the two diseases are quite different clinically, the immune dysfunction is quite similar—but the target is different. In multiple sclerosis, the body's immune system attacks the protective myelin covering of the nervous system, causing the many and varied neurological symptoms of MS, whereas in diabetes, the immune system attacks the pancreas. Nevertheless, investigators found a high level of similarity between the immunological reactions in both diseases. In fact, immune cells from people with diabetes attacked myelin proteins, and immune cells from people with MS attacked proteins in the pancreas! The researchers also found signs of abnormal immunity to cows' milk in the people in the study.

Gluten

Gluten is a protein found in a number of grain products including wheat, barley, rye, spelt and kamut. Celiac disease is a condition characterized by an allergy to this protein. Gluten sensitivity has been linked to a number of autoimmune conditions including type 1 diabetes. Children who were fed gluten before the age of four months have shown a significant increase in the chance of developing anti-pancreatic antibodies. Furthermore, celiac disease tends to increase the chances of an increased immune response to dairy products!

Recommendations

The intestinal tract is permeable to large molecules in the first months of life. Based on this and the information above, it is recommended that mothers breast-feed their infants and avoid exposing their children to cow's milk or gluten before one year of age. The protective effect of breastfeeding has now been documented for the autoimmune diseases Crohn's disease, ulcerative colitis, type 1 diabetes and celiac disease. Children at risk for diabetes, if they need to consume milk, should be given alternatives such as rice milk. Food introduction should focus on vegetables and fruits from age six months to one year. Only after the infant's first year should one consider introducing cow's milk, gluten, or any other foods that may induce allergy. Comprehensive IgE and IgG allergy testing, available from most naturopathic physicians, can help parents to design a diet specific to their child.

Vitamin D Deficiency

Vitamin D is a fat-soluble vitamin obtained naturally from two sources, exposure to sunlight and dietary consumption. Vitamin D3 (cholecalciferol) is the form of vitamin D produced in the skin and consumed in the diet. Another form of vitamin D, known as vitamin D2 (ergocalciferol), is produced by irradiating fungi, and is a much less effective and potentially more toxic source of vitamin D. Therefore, supplemental vitamin D should be taken in the form of vitamin D3 as opposed to vitamin D2. Other acceptable sources of vitamin D (other than cow's milk fortified with vitamin D) include fish liver oil, egg yolks, butter, liver and some fortified breakfast cereals. However, of these, fish liver oils seem to be the only source containing therapeutic amounts.

Exposure to UV rays found in sunlight enables the body to manufacture vitamin D. But this is only true at certain times of the year in climates that are distant from the equator. For example, in Boston no vitamin D is produced from sun exposure from October through March. This means that the body must rely on vitamin D stored in summer through out these months unless a supplement is taken. Yet based on advice from public health officials, many people cover up or use strong sun screens or sun blocks throughout the summer. The result is that vitamin D status, which can be measured in the blood with a 25-hydroxy vitamin D test, is often inadequate. Confounding this situation is that the RDA levels set for vitamin D may be too low to correct this widespread deficiency.

How are vitamin D levels connected to type 1 diabetes? Originally believed to influence only calcium absorption and bone density, it is now apparent that vitamin D plays an important role in immune system modulation. In a number of scientific studies, it has been found that low vitamin D levels increase the chances of getting type 1 diabetes. For example, in a study of more than 12,000 infants in Finland, it was found that the addition of 2,000 IU/day of vitamin D in infancy was associated with over an 80 percent decrease in the frequency of type 1 diabetes by age 30. It was also noted that children with rickets (weak bones due to vitamin D deficiency) during the first year of life had three times the chance of developing diabetes, compared with those children without rickets. The authors conclude that "ensuring adequate vitamin D supplementation for infants could help to reverse the increasing trend in the incidence of type 1 diabetes." Compare this to the US RDA of 200 IU of vitamin D/day for children and 400 IU/day for adults. In the Finnish study infants supplemented with less than 2,000 IU did better than those not supplemented at all, but not as well as those receiving the full dose. Note that vitamin D therapy should only be undertaken with the guidance of a healthcare practitioner familiar with its use.

Avoid Chemical Exposures

Evidence has been accumulating that exposure to a variety of chemicals can contribute to the development of both type 1 and type 2 diabetes. This is not surprising given that many chemicals have been shown to damage or destroy pancreatic beta cells or adversely affect insulin sensitivity. For instance, exposure to Agent Orange has been shown to increase diabetes rates by five percent. Agent Orange has been found in the tissues of 76 percent of the population of the United States. A number of research papers have also pointed to a connection between dioxin and/ or PCB occupational exposure and increased rates of diabetes. However, even non-occupational exposures may be putting the general public at risk. Exposure to these "background" levels of toxins may very likely increase the risk of diabetes in the general population.

Avoid Nitrates

Nitrates, which are added to cured meats such as hot dogs, cold cuts, and smoked fish, and are found in agricultural run-off, are also linked to the development of type 1 diabetes. There is an association between increased exposure to nitrates (from agricultural water contamination or from preservatives in food) and the development of type 1 diabetes. Nitrate-free food alternatives are available in health food stores. Water consumed should be purified and nitrate free. Nitrates, as well as contributing to diabetes by damaging the pancreas, have also been shown to be carcinogenic and to contribute to birth defects. The young are particularly at risk from exposure to these harmful chemicals.

Type 2 Prevention

According to the National Institute of Health, the risk factors for developing type 2 diabetes are:

- Advancing age

- Overweight

- Having a parent, brother, or sister with diabetes

- Family background that is Alaska Native, American Indian, African

- American, Hispanic/Latino American, Asian American, or Pacific Islander

- History of gestational diabetes, or having given birth to at least one baby weighing more than nine pounds

- Blood pressure 140/90 mm Hg or higher

- Cholesterol levels abnormal

- Inactive lifestyle and exercise fewer than three times a week

- Polycystic ovary syndrome, also called PCOS (women only)

- On previous testing, evidence of impaired glucose tolerance (IGT) or impaired fasting glucose (IFG) detected

- History of cardiovascular disease

How Did the Epidemic of Type 2 Diabetes Happen?

It has been estimated that an average hunter/gatherer existence requires the expenditure of 5000 to 6000 calories per day. A typical person in industrialized society burns 2000 to 3000 calories per day of energy. In addition, traditional food sources for the hunter/gatherer have been shown to be much more nutrient dense and to provide many times the current RDA (recommended daily allowance) levels for most vitamins and minerals. Grains were first cultivated in the Tigris/Euphrates region approximately 15,000 years ago. Before the cultivation of grains, humans and pre-humans survived on a hunter/gatherer diet of plants and animal protein. Hence, our genetic make-up has been fine-tuned over eons for a hunter/gatherer type lifestyle, as opposed to a modern high-calorie, high-carbohydrate, low-activity one.

One of the highest-risk groups for diabetes in North America is the aboriginal community. In some aboriginal communities obesity rates are up to 50 percent higher than the North American average, which is already unacceptably high. Diabetes rates show the same alarming trend. Fortunately, many native groups are now promoting traditional diets, increased activity levels and the use of traditional foods. For aboriginals, cutting down on carbohydrates isn't so much the latest fad diet as it is modern version of the traditional diet eaten by their ancestors for thousands of years.

Treatment Options for Diabetic Peripheral Neuropathy

A Healthy Person with Diabetes Diet

Although many factors such as stress, exercise, and the use of stimulants can affect blood sugar control, food is the most crucial concern for most persons with diabetes. The wrong diet can raise blood sugar levels sharply and often, immediately after its consumption. Given that we live in a society in which the wrong foods are not only abundantly available, but also widely promoted in advertising, the significance of a dietary approach to diabetes management cannot be overstated. In order to better manage blood sugar levels, reduce the risk of long-term diabetic complications, and enhance the potential to protect the body from free-radical damage, persons with diabetes need to follow a dietary program that manages food intake. This will not only enhance the body's ability to maintain healthy blood sugar levels, but also provide the optimum ability to heal the increased damage to tissues which is found in diabetes.

The recommended diet focuses on the consumption of low-glycemic index and low-glycemic load foods, with an emphasis on fresh fruits and vegetables and quality protein and fats. The approach offers the possibility of best controlling blood sugar levels while optimally nourishing the body. The glycemic index is simply a method of evaluating the speed at which certain foods can increase blood sugar after their consumption. One way to look at this approach is from a "good" carbohydrate versus a "bad" carbohydrate point of view. Good carbohydrates are lower on the glycemic index (less than 50), whereas bad carbohydrates are high on the glycemic index. Glycemic load is another way to measure whether a carbohydrate is classified as "good" versus "bad." Glycemic load takes into account not only the quality of the carbohydrate but also the quantity of carbohydrate in a particular food. As with glycemic index, a lower value is better for glycemic load. Tables of foods with their glycemic indices and loads are available on many Web sites and in the book *Healing Diabetes* (CCNM Press 2007), which also contains recipes and lists of specific foods which are beneficial for persons with diabetes. In general, for the optimal management of diabetes, no foods should be consumed with a glycemic index higher than 50. Consuming high-fiber foods, supplemental fiber, or protein with meals tends to modulate the glycemic index of foods, so this is encouraged.

When one examines the glycemic index chart, this diet may at first seem overly restrictive, especially considering modern day food processing techniques. Foods that would typically be restricted on a low GI diet include:

- Simple sugars and carbohydrates (sucrose, fructose, sweets, cookies, candy, ice cream, pastries, honey, fruit juice, soda pop, and alcoholic beverages, etc.)

- Refined grains and carbohydrates (white flour products such as white bread, white pasta, white rice, etc.)

- Most processed grain products (breads, pasta, cornbread, tortillas, crackers, popcorn, etc.)

These foods, however, were simply not available for most of the time during which the human metabolic system was evolving. This is illustrated by the fact that certain indigenous groups of people, who made the transition from a low glycemic "hunter/ gatherer" type diet to a diet high in refined carbohydrates very rapidly, have the highest rates of diabetes in the world. Many indigenous cultures relied on hunting and gathering techniques, and possibly farmed some fruits and vegetables. The transition to a life of reduced physical activity and a diet high in processed foods caused the number of diabetes cases within their population to explode. Researchers have hypothesized that this has occurred because their genes are "thrifty;" they are genetically programmed to maximize their energy storage from available calories. In other words, in the presence of refined carbohydrates, their thrifty genes lead to maximize fat storage. This elevates their blood sugar levels, which ultimately leads to the development of diabetes. Intervention programs designed to alter their diet and lifestyle to reflect their traditional life have been shown to dramatically improve blood sugar levels, even in those diagnosed with type 2 diabetes.

A low-glycemic diet is healthy for most people, no matter the condition of their health. Low-glycemic diets have been shown to reduce inflammation, support a healthy immune system, and may even slow the aging process. Many people have also found that the general principles of this dietary program are paramount for weight loss and long-term weight management.

Dietary Goals

No general diet can be precise for every individual. The goal of a healthy diet and supplement regime for persons with diabetes, whether type 1 or type 2, is a glycosylated hemoglobin (HbA1c) blood test level below 6 or, at least, between 6 and 7. This is the level that minimizes the long-term complications of diabetes. The equivalent goal in terms of glucose self-monitoring would be a fasting glucose (first thing in the morning) below 120 mg/dl (6.7 *mmol/L*) and 140 mg/dl (7.7 *mmol/L*) for readings taken two hours after eating. For many people, this may involve lowering glycemic index and load in stages until these goals are met. In other words, one can eliminate the highest glycemic foods first, and then refine the diet in stages until the goal is met. For example, one person may be able to eat foods with a glycemic load of 50 three times per day to achieve good blood sugar control, whereas another may have to limit carbohydrate foods to only a glycemic load of 30 per meal. Of course, other lifestyle factors such as exercise, stress and nutritional status (the level of vitamins and minerals in the cells) will influence the results obtained with diet. Nevertheless, a good starting point would be a goal of glycemic load of 150 per day total or less.

Allergen Free

More and more research has linked inflammation in the body to a wide range of degenerative medical conditions, including heart disease, diabetes, cancer, Alzheimer's and Parkinson's. One simple way to reduce inflammation is to identify and then avoid foods that trigger an inflammatory response. Allergy tests are now readily available from many healthcare providers, including naturopathic doctors, who can assess food allergies from a simple blood test called IgG/IgE ELISA testing. Some of the more common allergenic foods include dairy products, gluten (found in some grains, such as wheat), eggs, citrus and soy. Keep in mind however that everyone is different and the foods that may be healthy for one person may make another ill. In clinical practice it is evident that the avoidance of allergenic foods can result in remarkable benefits in terms of energy, immune function, weight management, as well as blood sugar control. Once again these recommendations apply not only to persons with diabetes but to anyone with chronic disease or just interested in optimal health.

Nutrient Excesses and Deficiencies Coexist in North America

It has been said that North Americans suffer predominantly from diseases of excess. This is only partly true, in that along with the excesses (of refined sugars and carbohydrates) come deficiencies. The processed foods and fast foods many people eat regularly not only have an excess of "empty" calories, they also require more nutrients just to help our bodies digest them! These processed foods can actually deplete the level of health-giving nutrients in our bodies by damaging these nutrients or increasing their excretion from the body. In addition, many food additives, environmental toxins and pharmaceutical drugs have also been shown to contribute to nutrient deficiency. Add to that equation the constant depletion of nutrients from our soils by industrial agriculture and we have a recipe for widespread nutrient deficiency in North America. If diabetes is indeed a disease of nutrient deficiency, resulting in poor carbohydrate metabolism, as some experts believe, then it would make sense that correcting these deficiencies before too much damage is done may reverse type 2 diabetes. The good news is that this is more often than not the case; type 2 diabetes can often be reversed.

> "In 1821, the average intake of sugar was 10 lbs./ year. Today it is 170 lbs., which is one quarter of the caloric intake. Another large portion of total calories comes from white flour and refined vegetable oils. Therefore, less than half our diet must provide all nutrients to a body that is under constant stress from its intake of sugar, white flour, rancid and hydrogenated oils. This, then, can be seen as the root cause of the vast increase in degenerative diseases that plague modern America."
>
> – Sally Fallon and Mary Enig, Nourishing Traditions

Therefore, although the total caloric intake in the diet of many North Americans is generally well above adequate levels, the diet is deficient in many nutrients. These nutrients, such as magnesium, chromium, B-vitamins, vitamin E, all mentioned below, are required for healthy people to prevent diabetes, and for persons with diabetes to maintain or improve their current health. Persons with diabetes especially need to eat a nutrient-dense diet to minimize or prevent the damage from free radicals caused by their faulty metabolism. Free radicals are neutralized in the body by antioxidants, such as vitamin C, vitamin E, selenium and bioflavonoids. Free radical production is magnified for anyone dealing with diabetes. Thus, it is crucial for persons with diabetes to receive high levels of antioxidants, both in their foods and in the form of supplements.

Sugar Cravings

Sugar cravings should be taken quite seriously as they can be very powerful and can sabotage the efforts of the most dedicated. Sugar is a very addictive substance, a fact which has been proven in a number of research trials in mammals. In humans, sugar cravings that last for more than one week on a low glycemic diet (the first week should be considered "sugar withdrawal") are often associated with disease conditions and nutrient deficiencies or imbalances. For instance, chronic fungal infections such as candida albicans in the gastrointestinal tract, vagina, or skin can contribute to sugar cravings. Other chronic infections may also be responsible and investigated. An imbalance of protein and carbohydrate in the diet or even in a particular meal may result in sugar cravings right after eating. Nutrient deficiencies, such as vitamin and mineral deficiencies, may also contribute to sugar cravings. Finally, chronic stress and weakened adrenal glands can result in low blood sugar between meals (hypoglycemia), which will result in very strong sugar cravings. Any or all of the above scenarios requires addressing or it will be very difficult to maintain a low glycemic diet with sheer will power.

A Word About Grains

Grains, such as wheat, rye and oats are neither "bad" nor "good" carbohydrates. They must be classified by their glycemic index and glycemic load like all other foods. Since grains are mostly carbohydrate, it is easy to see how their over-consumption can contribute to obesity and diabetes, especially if they are processed as opposed to "whole." Processing strips nutrients and fiber from the grain, which inherently raises the glycemic index. It also often makes the grain more readily converted by the body into glucose. "Quick" oats and "converted" rice are examples of processed grains which are higher than their less-refined versions on the glycemic scale. Eating refined grains may also help to create food cravings and result in mood swings. Following a meal of high glycemic grains, people with insulin resistance or type 2 diabetes will find their blood glucose levels rising quickly, stimulating the pancreas to release insulin in order to lower blood sugar levels. Insulin in the blood sends a message to store this high-carbohydrate meal as fat. Insulin blocks glucagon, a hormone which promotes the burning of fat and sugar. Insulin also blocks the production of human growth hormone, important in many vital bodily functions, including helping to build muscle and to sleep well. The net result is that over-consumption of especially refined grains can lead to increased fat storage, decreased fat burning, weight gain and eventually diabetes.

Detrimental Effects of High Insulin Levels

- Cravings shortly following a meal

- Higher blood pressure

- Higher triglycerides and lower good (HDL) cholesterol

- Weight gain that is difficult to lose by dieting

- Increased risk of heart attack and stroke

- Depletion of important nutrients

- Increased incidence of osteoporosis

- Increased risk of type 2 diabetes

- Increased inflammation and immune dysfunction

Table 2: Detrimental Effects of High Insulin Levels

Good and Bad Fats

The food industry in North America has for a long time been obsessed with fat. "Low fat" products have sprouted all over supermarket shelves. Unfortunately, sugar often replaces the fat in these foods, and as discussed, sugar is easily converted to fat by the body for storage. Hence, during the "low fat" revolution, obesity rates skyrocketed. North Americans are finally hearing more and more these days about the benefits of "good" fats, and the dangers of "bad" fats. These good fats include monounsaturated and polyunsaturated and fats, and exclude most saturated fats and all human-made trans fats (created through the chemical processing and hydrogenation of otherwise unsaturated fats). The terms "omega-3" and "omega-6" fatty acids are now commonly seen in all sorts of products, ranging from health supplements (mentioned below in the supplement section) to eggs and even milk.

The importance of fat in the diet is connected to the use of fats by the body. Fats eaten in the diet are incorporated into the cell membranes. Healthy cell membranes allow the cell to control the contents inside the cell versus outside the cell. Leaky or damaged cell membranes, made with inferior fats, will allow toxins and free radicals to enter the cells and important nutrients to leak out. Even insulin receptors and the passage of insulin, as well as other hormones, such as thyroid hormone and adrenal hormones, are influenced by the health of the cell membranes. The right kinds of fats can even slow digestion and absorption of carbohydrates, thereby lessening the insulin reaction. Thus the importance of eating correct fats cannot be overemphasized for any healthy diet, but especially for the person with diabetes diet.

Trans fats are artificially created fats that increase the risk of diabetes. Their consumption has also been shown to increase the risk of other serious chronic diseases, including heart disease and cancer. Trans fats become a part of the cell and block the cell's utilization of "good" essential fatty acids, while interfering with insulin receptors. They raise the level of bad cholesterol more than animal (saturated) fats. Trans fats are often found in most fried or deep fried foods, most margarines, commercially-prepared snacks and baked goods, peanut butter, pastries, crackers, cookies, pies, and cakes. These fats should be totally avoided by everyone as they are not safe for consumption. More than 1 gram per day increases the risk of cardiovascular disease; the typical teenager in our society eats 35 grams per day of trans fats!

Essential fatty acids (EFAs) are considered the "good" fats of human nutrition. These are fats that the body needs and so they must be obtained from the diet. Essential fatty acids are needed for the health of many tissues in the body including the heart, eyes, skin, digestive system, immune system, joints, and brain. They also help fight insulin resistance, lower triglycerides, normalize blood pressure, reduce inflammation, prevent blood clots, and decrease the risk of stroke, dementia, and Alzheimer's disease. Some experts in the field of nutrition now believe that a deficiency of EFAs is responsible for most of the chronic disease both physical and mental, seen in the western industrialized world.

There are two main types of EFAs known as omega-3 and omega-6. A healthy ratio of omega-6 to omega-3 EFAs is in the range of 4:1 to 1:1; however, the North American diet typically contains an unhealthy EFA ratio of 20-25:1 omega-6 to omega-3 fatty acids. Persons with diabetes need to eat fats and oils that address this imbalance. One way to do this is to increase the consumption of cold-water fish. This approach can only be recommended if a good source of mercury-free or low-mercury fish is available. Fish lower on the food chain, such as sardines and small mackerel, tend to be lower in mercury than fish like tuna and swordfish, which are typically higher in mercury. High quality cod liver oil in the winter and fish oil supplements may be better choices. Taking cod liver oil in the winter also helps to provide us with vitamin D. However, be sure to check that fish oil supplements are tested and guaranteed free of contaminants.

Another type of fat which needs to be avoided is saturated fat. This fat is found in higher amounts in most factory farmed meats and in regular-fat dairy products. Saturated fats are usually solid at room temperature. Too much saturated fat in the diet is considered unhealthy, and may contribute to the development of heart disease and diabetes. It is best to consume animal fats in moderation. This can be achieved for most people by choosing lean meats, chicken and turkey without the skin, and wild meats or free-range pasture-fed meats, which are generally leaner and provide a better fat profile than meat from grain-fed factory-farmed animals. Free-range pasture-fed livestock tends to contain higher levels of omega-3 fatty acids and conjugated linoleic acid (CLA), as well as other beneficial substances.

A final type of fat which is important in human nutrition is called omega-9 fatty acids. These fats tend to lower LDL, the "bad" cholesterol. Omega-9, also called monounsaturated oils, can be found in healthy foods such as extra virgin olive oil (unfiltered, cloudy, golden yellow) or cold-pressed macadamia nut oil. Omega-9 oils are also found in many nuts and seeds. Since omega-9 oils contain only one unsaturated bond, they tend to be more stable in cooking than polyunsaturated oils. Omega-9 oils such as olive oil are therefore recommended for sautéing.

Burning Feet in the Court Room

Barry, a 64-year-old lawyer complained of progressively worsening burning pain, tingling, and numbness of both feet. He had noticed this discomfort for a number of years and had ignored the symptoms, thinking that he had been tying his shoe laces too tight, a habit he developed in his early days in the military. He had been seen both by his family doctor and neurologist, who confirmed the diagnosis of peripheral neuropathy but offered no treatment or explanation as to the cause. Diabetes had been

*ruled out based on blood tests. Barry was finding that his pain
was now affecting his ability to focus on his work as a crown
prosecutor, which often required that he spend long days standing in court.*

*Other health concerns of Barry's included high blood pres-
sure, for which he was taking three medications—a diuretic, a
calcium channel blocker and an angiotensin inhibitor. He had
also been diagnosed with hypothyroidism years earlier for which
he was prescribed synthetic thyroid hormone. A recent angio-
gram revealed mild atherosclerosis, and Barry's cardiologist
found evidence of at least one silent heart attack.*

*Upon examination of Barry's recent blood work it was noted
that although blood sugar was in the normal range it was near
the upper end of that range. In addition, triglycerides were elevated and HDL (good cholesterol) was dangerously low. Combined with truncal obesity, high blood pressure, and an inactive
lifestyle, it was concluded that Barry's neuropathy was likely a
symptom of a form of "pre-diabetes" known as metabolic syndrome X.*

Treatment

*Barry was immediately put on a vitamin and mineral protocol in-
cluding 750 mcg per day of chromium, 600 mg per day of lipoic
acid, 1000 mg three times per day of evening primrose oil and an
herbal blood sugar-balancing formula. He was also counseled
in how to follow a low glycemic diet and agreed to slowly begin
an exercise program. He also began applying a topical natural
analgesic before bed to his feet.*

One month later Barry reported a 50 percent improvement in pain and a lessening of the total area of his feet that was affected. After two months, the left foot felt 100 percent normal with some intermittent numbness in the right foot, and by three months Barry reported no symptoms of neuropathy. Barry was very pleased and decided to continue with his new diet and supplements, having noted more energy as well. Six months after beginning this routine, a follow-up stress test showed no evidence of the previous heart damage. His blood pressure also had come down such that he was able to discontinue one of his medications and lower the doses of the others. Barry continues to do well, reporting only the occasional neuropathy sensations if he strays too far from the recommended diet – such as over Christmas holidays!

The Top 13 Supplements for Persons with Diabetec Peripheral Neuropathy

Lipoic Acid

Lipoic acid is a very much investigated nutrient for diabetic neuropathy, and for many it provided the first clear evidence that nutritional treatment can reverse the course of neuropathy. At least 15 controlled, randomized clinical trials of lipoic acid in patients with diabetic neuropathy have been done using different study designs, durations of treatment, doses, sample sizes, and patient populations. Also known as "alpha-lipoic acid," it is a powerful free radical scavenger found in the cells of humans and in a variety of foods. It has been called a "universal" antioxidant because it is both fat- and water-soluble, and it has also been shown to recycle other antioxidants, such as vitamins E and C. Lipoic acid has also been used to reverse damage associated with mushroom poisoning, radiation, alcoholic hepatitis, and heavy metal toxicity.

Lipoic acid is approved in Germany for clinical use in the management of diabetic polyneuropathy, and it has been used for this purpose in Europe for decades. A systematic review done in Germany of 15 trials concluded that short-term treatment with alpha-lipoic acid, 600 mg/day, reduces the symptoms of diabetic neuropathy. Statistically significant improvements in pain, tingling, and numbness compared with placebo were seen at this dose in a number of trials. Depletion of lipoic acid has also been documented in those with diabetic neuropathies. Research on lipoic acid supplementation has also shown improvements in glucose metabolism, reduced glycosylation of proteins (such as HbA1c), improved blood flow to peripheral nerves, and stimulation of nerve cell conduction. In one study, treatment with lipoic acid improved the efficiency with which insulin worked by 27 percent in only four weeks.

Clinical studies to date have indicated that alpha-lipoic acid is generally safe and well tolerated with minimal side effects. Adverse effects tend to be mild and include headache, skin rash, and stomach upset at high doses (>600 mg/day).

Methylcobalamin

Methylcobalamin is the active form of vitamin B12. Cyanocobalamin, another form of B12, is the most widely available and least expensive form of this B vitamin, and is found in most over-the-counter multivitamins. However, cyanocobalamin is an inactive precursor that must be converted into one of two active metabolites: methylcobalamin and adenosylcobalamin. Of these two, methylcobalamin seems to be the most neurologically active. Studies have suggested that methylcobalamin is better utilized by the body and better retained in tissue than cyanocobalamin. The clinical experience of many health care practitioners seems to further support the use of the methylcobalamin form for nerve-related conditions.

Vitamin B12 plays a critical role in the maintenance of nerve myelin, and it is well known that prolonged B12 deficiency in healthy individuals can lead to nerve degeneration and irreversible neurological damage. This is particularly a concern for persons with diabetes, since persons with diabetes have been shown to have lower B12 levels than healthy people. Furthermore, some diabetic medications such as metformin have been shown to deplete B12 levels. Supplementation of vitamin B12 in the form of methylcobalamin may benefit diabetic neuropathy by correcting a deficiency, as mentioned, or by protecting nerve fibers from degeneration. This protective effect was seen in animal studies, where supplementation of diabetic rats with methycobalamin protected nerve fibers from demyelination.

In one study of the effects of supplementation in humans, methylcobalamin was given to diabetic neuropathy sufferers for four months at a dose of 500 mcg, three times per day, taken orally. The treatment group showed statistical improvement in the symptoms of diabetic neuropathy, including burning sensation, numbness and pain, versus the placebo group. In another study, 20 type 2 persons with diabetes took supplements with 1,500 mcg/day methylcobalamin for two months. This resulted in improved vibration perception and improvement in heart rate variability (a sign of improvement in autonomic neuropathy) in the persons with diabetes group.

The recommended dosage for clinical effects in persons with diabetes is 5 to 15 mg per day (yes, milligrams) of methylcobalamin, taken orally (sublingually), intramuscularly or intravenously. Positive clinical results have been reported irrespective of the method of administration. Methylcobalamin has excellent tolerability and no known toxicity. Alcohol, antibiotics, oral hypoglycemic agents, beta blockers, anti-acid drugs (H2 blockers), oral contraceptives, nicotine, and HIV drugs can also cause vitamin B12 depletion.

Benfotiamine

Benfotiamine is a fat-soluble form of vitamin B1 (thiamine). B vitamin therapy has been used to treat neurological disorders such as diabetic neuropathy for many years. However, in 1954, Fujiwara discovered a group of fat-soluble thiamine derivatives, subsequently named allithiamines, because they occur naturally in allium family vegetables—garlic, onions, leeks, shallots, etc. Of these, benfotiamine seems to be the most effective. Benfotiamine, acting as a "super-charged" thiamine, helps maintain healthy cells in the presence of excess blood glucose. Oral administration of benfotiamine has been shown to raise thiamine levels in blood and tissues as much as four to five times higher than the water-soluble version. Benfotiamine exerts its beneficial effects by inhibiting all three major biochemical pathways implicated in diabetes-induced damage; the hexosamine pathway, the diaglycerol-protein kinase C pathway, and the formation of advanced glycation end products (AGEs). Benfotiamine does this by stimulating transketolase, a cellular enzyme essential for maintenance of normal glucose metabolic pathways. As such, benfotiamine, in addition to showing effectiveness against diabetic neuropathy, has also been shown to be valuable in the treatment of diabetic retinopathy and nephropathy.

In one double-blind, placebo-controlled study, 20 subjects with diabetic neuropathy were given 400 mg of benfotiamine daily for three weeks while another 20 subjects received placebo. In the treatment group a statistically significant improvement in the neuropathy score was reported compared to placebo, with a decrease in pain being the most significant improvement reported. In another trial, 24 people suffering with diabetic neuropathy took either benfotiamine (plus doses of common vitamin B6 and B12 similar to those used in mutivitamins) or a placebo, for 12 weeks. The benfotiamine treatment group started with 320 mg of benfotiamine per day for the first two weeks, followed by 120 mg per day for the rest of the trial. At the end of the trial, the vibration perception had improved by 30 percent in those who had taken the benfotiamine supplements, while it had worsened in the placebo group. People taking benfotiamine also experienced a statistically significant improvement in nerve conduction velocity from the feet, while this measurement also deteriorated in the placebo group. No adverse events were reported.

In general, studies of benfotiamine have shown improvements in pain, vibration sense, and nerve conduction. Significant improvements in these measurements are often seen by the third week of the trials. Also, when benfotiamine is used at lower doses the effects seem less pronounced. The most typical effective doses for benfotiamine are in the range of 300 to 400 mg per day in divided doses. Overall, benfotiamine users have reported a remarkable 50 to 88 percent reduction in diabetic nerve pain, depending on the dosage used and the study length.

Several studies have investigated the effect of benfotiamine in combination with multi-B vitamins, or compared to other B vitamins, in the treatment of diabetic neuropathy. In patients receiving the conventional B vitamin treatment, slight improvements in neuropathy symptoms have been noted, but typically not as remarkable as when combined with benfotiamine. Since benfotiamine has also shown promise for the treatment and prevention of retinal damage and kidney damage, with no reports of toxicity or safety issues, it is a highly recommended supplement for persons with diabetes.

Chromium

Awareness of chromium as a trace element in human nutrition began in 1929 when it was discovered that brewer's yeast (which is high in chromium) increased the blood sugar-lowering effects of insulin therapy. Deficiency of chromium has since been linked to a number of disorders, including decreased glucose tolerance and type 2 diabetes. Chromium exists in three forms, and it is nutritional chromium (also known as chromium III) which is found in foods and supplements. Other forms of chromium do not give a therapeutic benefit and are potentially toxic. It is believed that nutritional chromium increases the effectiveness of insulin as a cofactor in a molecule known as "glucose tolerance factor." Some have even postulated that insulin-resistant diabetes is a disease of chromium deficiency. This is supported by a number of documented human cases in which parenteral nutrition (feeding with a tube) have resulted in low chromium levels, high blood sugar levels, and even diabetic complications, such as neuropathy. Research has shown that chromium supplementation at 250 ug/day reversed these problems, including the neuropathies.

A number of clinical studies have also looked at blood sugar, insulin levels and chromium. Many of these studies have demonstrated that chromium is effective in treating both types of diabetes. One controlled study of 180 type 2 persons with diabetes involved random supplementation of placebo, 200 mcg chromium, or 1000 mcg of chromium (as chromium picolinate) every day over a period of four months. Fasting and two-hour post-glucose consumption blood sugar levels were measured. Blood sugar levels decreased significantly in the 1000 mcg group, while the 200 mcg group had no significant drop. As well, after four months, nearly all of the diabetes patients in the higher dose group no longer had symptoms of diabetes. Their blood sugar and insulin levels dropped to near normal. It should be noted that this is an achievement rarely seen with pharmaceutical diabetes medications.

In another study, 162 persons with diabetes (48 type 1 diabetes, 114 type 2) were given 200 mcg of chromium picolinate daily. 71 percent of the type 1 patients responded positively with an overall 30 percent decrease of their insulin dose. Thus, even persons with diabetes who inject insulin and/or are in the later stages of diabetes respond positively to chromium supplementation. Many persons with diabetes have trouble with good blood sugar control. Chromium supplementation in this study resulted in improved blood sugar control as quickly as 10 days after the beginning of treatment!

The recommended daily intake (RDI) for chromium is 50 to 200 mcg of chromium per day. Unfortunately, the majority of North Americans do not get even the minimum RDI of many nutrients, including chromium, from their diets. This lack of chromium may be contributing to the epidemic of diabetes. It may be reasonable for the average healthy person with no personal or family history of diabetes to supplement with the RDI amounts of chromium, but higher amounts are likely needed for people with conditions involving insulin resistance and blood sugar control problems, such as type 1 diabetes, type 2 diabetes, or insulin resistance/pre-diabetes. In clinical trials diabetes patients who have taken 200 mcg per day of chromium have had some slight improvement in their condition in the longer term. Those who took 1000 mcg per day, however, had faster and more pronounced results. It also seems that patients with type 2 diabetes and insulin resistance/syndrome X have greater excretion of chromium, lower tissue levels of chromium, and less of an ability to utilize chromium in the body.

Toxicity of chromium has been associated with the chromium VI (non-nutritional) form. Nutritional chromium (III) is found naturally in many foods, and nutritional supplements are available in various complex forms, such as picolinate, polynicotinate, and citrate. The use of 1000 mcg/day chromium as picolinate in type 2 diabetic patients for a period of four months showed no toxicity. Chromium therapy should be undertaken with the guidance of a healthcare practitioner familiar with its use.

Vanadium

Vanadium is a trace mineral which has been used for the control of blood sugar even prior to the discovery of insulin. Evidence suggests that vanadium supports vital metabolic processes because of its ability to mimic the actions of insulin. Numerous human and animal studies have shown that vanadium supplementation can improve fasting glucose and other measures of diabetes. In addition, in animal models, vanadium appears to decrease appetite and body weight in insulin-resistant animals.

A number of small human studies have shown that vanadium is effective at improving insulin sensitivity. In one placebo-controlled study, eight subjects with type 2 diabetes received 50 mg vanadyl sulfate twice daily for four weeks. Improvements in fasting glucose and insulin resistance were documented. In another trial, 100 mg of vanadyl sulfate given daily for three weeks decreased fasting plasma glucose and improved insulin sensitivity in diabetic subjects. In another trial, 11 type 2 diabetic patients were treated with vanadium sulfate at a higher dose (150 mg/day) and for a longer period of time (six weeks). Treatment with vanadium significantly improved glycemic control, and fasting glucose decreased from an average of 194 to 155 mg/dL, and hemoglobin A1c decreased from an average of 8.1 to 7.6.

Absorption of dietary vanadium and supplemental vanadium sulfate is poor. Studies show that less than 5 percent of dietary vanadium is absorbed. Organic forms of vanadium, such as bis-glycinato oxovanadium (BGOV), are recognized as being more absorbable. BGOV is an organically bound, bio-available form of vanadium composed with the amino acid glycine. Absorption is in the range of approximately 50 percent, with reduced chances of the gastrointestinal side effects sometimes seen with vanadium sulfate supplementation. The daily dietary intake in humans has been estimated to vary from 10 mcg to 2 mg of elemental vanadium, depending on the environmental sources. In animals, vanadium has been shown to be an essential mineral. More research on vanadium is needed to establish an accurate dose/response for the treatment of insulin resistance. However, based on current evidence, doses of vanadium from organic sources in the range of 1 to 10 mg/day short term (up to one month) and 0.5 to 2 mg/day long term seem reasonable. Vanadium therapy should only be undertaken with the guidance of a health care practitioner familiar with its use.

Vitamin E

Oxidative stress (free radical damage) appears to play a significant role in the development of the complications of diabetes, including peripheral neuropathy. Vitamin E is an antioxidant which protects cells from free radical damage. Diets high in vitamin E have been shown to be protective against many health conditions, including diabetes. Vitamin E can benefit persons with diabetes by not only protecting vulnerable nerve tissue, but also protecting small blood vessels, improving circulation, and reducing the negative effects of LDL cholesterol. It is important, however, to get the right form of vitamin E. The best forms are known as "natural, mixed tocopherol" forms of vitamin E which contains a variety of naturally occurring vitamin E molecules designated as "d " as in "d-alpha tocopherol." Avoid synthetic forms which are labeled "dl" as in "dl-alpha tocopherol."

In terms of peripheral neuropathy, vitamin E was studied in a double-blind, placebo-controlled trial of 21 type 2 persons with diabetic peripheral neuropathy. They were given either 900 mg vitamin E or placebo for six months. Electrophysiological measurements of nerve function significantly improved in two of 12 parameters tested, including nerve conduction, in the vitamin E group compared to placebo. In another study which looked at diabetic rats, depletion of vitamin E resulted in nerve conduction problems similar to those seen in people with diabetic neuropathy. Therefore it is recommended that persons with diabetes take 400 to 800 IU per day of natural, mixed tocopherol form vitamin E.

Vitamin D

As previously mentioned, low circulating vitamin D levels are associated with the development of type 1 diabetes, and supplementation of vitamin D in infancy has been shown to reduce the risk of developing this type of diabetes by 80 percent. Vitamin D also seems to play a role in the maintenance of healthy blood sugar levels in healthy individuals, type 2 persons with diabetes, and those with insulin resistance. For instance, in one study, healthy adults with higher serum vitamin D levels had significantly lower 60-minute, 90-minute, and 120-minute postprandial (after eating) glucose levels and better insulin sensitivity than those who were vitamin D-deficient. It was noted by the study authors that vitamin D outperformed the common oral diabetic pharmaceutical medication metformin. Those with the highest vitamin D status had an improvement of insulin sensitivity of 60 percent, versus a 13 percent improvement typical with metformin.

Another clinical trial used 1332 IU per day of vitamin D for only 30 days in 10 women with type 2 diabetes. This relatively modest level of vitamin D supplementation over a short period was shown to improve insulin sensitivity by a remarkable 21 percent. More and more evidence is now pointing to the likelihood that the typical dosage of vitamin D used in supplements, and based on the RDA values, falls far short of optimal levels. Consider that full-body exposure to ultraviolet light can produce 10,000 to 25,000 IU of vitamin D3 per day, which is much higher than the RDA. Also recall that the dose of 2,000 IU used to prevent type 1 diabetes in infants is 10 times the RDA, yet no negative effects were noted. It is also likely that the majority of studies in adults have used inadequate doses of vitamin D and that is why they may have failed to identify therapeutic benefits from vitamin D supplementation. A more reasonable vitamin D dose for adult studies may be 5,000 to 10,000 IU per day, continued for at least three to four months until vitamin D levels plateau. A blood test for 25-hydroxy-vitamin D can ascertain whether vitamin D levels have reached an optimum level. Vitamin D therapy should, however, only be undertaken with the guidance of a healthcare practitioner familiar with its use.

Multi-B Vitamins

Considering that the B vitamin group affects many aspects of cell metabolism and therefore healthy nerve functioning, it may be more effective to supplement the entire group of B vitamins.

As mentioned in the benfotiamine section, benfotiamine has been combined with other B vitamins in some of the diabetic neuropathy trials with good results. For example, in one study, 30 patients received 50 mg benfotiamine and 250 mcg B12 (as cyanocobalamin per tablet) at a dose of two tablets four times daily for three weeks, for a total daily dose of 400 mg benfotiamine and 2,000 mcg B12, followed by one tablet three times daily for nine weeks. The second group of 15 subjects received a B-complex vitamin supplement at a dose of two tablets three times daily for the entire three months. All the patients received benefit, but the group taking befotiamine had significant relief of symptoms versus a slight improvement for the multi-B group.

However, a combination of B1, B6 and B12 was tested in an animal model of neuropathic pain. In this case, recovery from pain was rated as 20 to 100 percent at 12 hours, with recovery being twice as fast as a saline (salt) placebo. Overall, the B vitamin combination reduced both the severity and duration of pain. The authors concluded: "These results strongly support the clinical use of B vitamins in aiding the treatment of chronic pain and/or other diseases due to similar injuries to the nervous system." In these animal studies, results were likely more pronounced than in the human multi-B vitamin trials due to the fact that the neuropathy was induced immediately prior to treatment, as opposed to typical diabetic neuropathy in humans which takes years to develop and typically is present long before treatment is initiated. Nevertheless, including a multiple B vitamin seems a prudent approach to maximizing the potential for nerve repair, especially for anyone taking pharmaceutical drugs for pain, which are known to deplete B vitamin levels.

Gymnema

Gymnema (*gymnema sylvestre*) is a plant from India that has been used traditionally for the treatment of diabetes. Human clinical trials have shown that gymnema sylvestre is useful for treating both type 1 and type 2 diabetes. The first scientific confirmation of gymnema's use in diabetes came almost 70 years ago when it was demonstrated that gymnema reduced urine glucose in persons with diabetes. More recently, in diabetic rats, fasting blood glucose levels returned to normal after 60 days of gymnema with oral administration. The therapy led to a rise in serum insulin to levels closer to normal fasting levels. In the diabetic rat pancreas, gymnema was able to double the number of insulin-producing cells.

In a more recent human trial, both type 1 and 2 persons with diabetes were given a standardized gymnema leaf extract for a period of two years. Insulin requirements were decreased by about one-half in the 27 type 1 persons with diabetes in the study, and the average blood glucose decreased from 232 mg/dL to 152 mg/dL. Glycosylated plasma protein levels also decreased. Serum lipids also returned to normal levels with gymnema therapy. Most impressively, an increase in C-peptide levels were found, which is a strong indication of increased insulin production. Type 2 diabetic patients on conventional oral anti-hyperglycemic agents also have shown improvement with gymnema. During supplementation, type 2 patients showed a significant reduction in blood glucose, glycosylated hemoglobin, and glycosylated plasma proteins. Conventional oral hypoglycemic drug dosage was decreased, and five of 22 diabetic patients were able to discontinue their conventional drug treatment altogether and maintain their blood glucose homeostasis with gymnema sylves-

tre alone. Additionally, gymnema significantly improved cholesterol, triglyceride, and free fatty acid levels that were previously
elevated.

The typical therapeutic dose of gymnema for treatment of
diabetes, standardized to contain 24 percent gymnemic acids, is
400 to 600 mg daily. In adult-onset persons with diabetes, ongo-
ing use for periods as long as two years has proven successful.
Because it acts gradually, gymnema extract should be consumed
regularly with meals for several days/weeks and can be taken for
months/years with no significant side effects. However, patients
taking gymnema may require dosage adjustments of other antidi-
abetic drugs, and therefore treatment should be undertaken with
the guidance of a health care professional familiar with its use.

Jambul

Jambul is a traditional treatment for diabetes native to southern
Asia, India, Indonesia, and Australia. The seed is considered
to be one of the most powerful hypoglycemic agents in the
Ayurvedic repertory. In India, as little as one teaspoon per day of
ground seed was a traditional treatment for type 2 diabetes. In a
number of animal studies, jambul has been shown to have blood
sugar-lowering and cholestrol-lowering effects. "Jamboline,"
a component of jambul, is believed to inhibit the conversion
of starch into glucose, thereby helping to balance blood sugar
levels. The recommended dose of jambul is 800 mg per meal in
capsule form.

Essential Fatty Acids

There are two essential fatty acids in human nutrition: omega-3 and omega-6. They are often consumed in the diet as linolenic and linoleic acid. However, these fatty acids require an enzyme called delta-6 desaturase to convert into their useful forms. Delta-6 desaturase converts linolenic acid to eicosapentaenoic acid (EPA) and linoleic acid to gamma-linoleic acid (GLA). This conversion process is often severely compromised in persons with diabetes. Metabolites of GLA are essential for nerve membrane structure and healthy circulation, and thus a deficiency could contribute to the development of neuropathy. Therefore, persons with diabetes need to be particularly careful about selecting good dietary sources of essential fatty acids, and balancing them properly. Even so, it is recommended that persons with diabetes supplement their diet with the two pre-converted essential fatty acids mentioned: EPA (typically from fish oils) and GLA (from evening primrose, black currant, or borage oils). Note that, while flaxseed oil is often recommended as a good fat because it contains high amounts of omega-3 EFAs, it is only utilized properly if insulin and blood sugar levels are well managed and nutrient cofactors are present in adequate amounts. Therefore, flax oil is generally not the best choice for persons with diabetes as a source of omega-3 fatty acids.

The importance of supplemental essential fatty acids in persons with diabetes has been investigated in at least two clinical trials. In one double-blind study, 22 patients with diabetic neuropathy were assigned to receive 360 mg GLA or placebo for six months. People who took the GLA exhibited significantly better neuropathy symptoms and nerve impulse measurements compared to the placebo group. In another study, the effect of

GLA on diabetic neuropathy patients in London was investigated over a one-year period. One hundred and eleven subjects with mild diabetic neuropathy were given either GLA or a placebo. By measuring 16 different parameters, the researchers concluded that significant beneficial effects were detectable in offering GLA to persons with diabetes with neuropathy. Although the research techniques used in these studies have been called into question, a number of animal studies have supported the results. In diabetic rats, supplementation with 260 mg GLA daily, either at onset of diabetes for 12 weeks (preventive group) or after six weeks of diabetes for six weeks (reversal group), resulted in restoration of normal nerve function in both the prevention and reversal groups. Another animal study found GLA improves nerve function and blood flow to the nerves, whether the GLA came from evening primrose oil or other sources, indicating that the benefit is from GLA as opposed to other ingredients found in evening primrose.

Omega-3 fatty acids are also essential for healthy nerve cell function and blood flow. A clinical study of 21 type 2 persons with diabetic peripheral neuropathy found that 1,800 mg EPA per day for 48 weeks significantly decreased symptoms such as numbness and improved proprioception. Blood flow to the feet and cholesterol levels also significantly improved. In animals, a study in diabetic rats found fish oil, compared to olive oil, increased nerve conduction and prevented nerve damage. Researchers have also studied DHA, a related omega-3 fatty acid, and also found benefits in animal models of diabetes. It is therefore recommended that persons with diabetes supplement with an EPA/DHA blend at a daily dose of 1,800 mg of EPA and 900 mg DHA.

Magnesium

The common mineral magnesium is an essential cofactor in human metabolism, assisting more than 300 chemical reactions including the conversion of glucose to energy. Magnesium deficiency has been associated with high blood pressure, diabetes, high cholesterol, cardiovascular disease, and complications of pregnancy. Decreased magnesium levels and increased losses of magnesium in the urine have been documented in both type 1 and type 2 diabetics. In addition, the use of certain medications, including diuretics for high blood pressure, can deplete magnesium. Malabsorption syndromes of the gastrointestinal tract, low stomach acid (hypochlorhydria), diets low in minerals, and alcohol and caffeine use can also cause magnesium depletion.

Studies of magnesium supplementation have shown a positive effect on insulin sensitivity and triglyceride levels, but mixed results in terms of blood sugar control. However, studies have demonstrated that magnesium supplementation may help to prevent type 2 diabetes. In one study, the protective aspect of magnesium was examined by the effect of magnesium supplementation on obese rats over a period of six weeks. By the end of the study period, all of the control animals became diabetic, while only one of the eight rats in the magnesium supplementation group developed the disease. By preventing deterioration of glucose tolerance, magnesium may thus delay or prevent type 2 diabetes. In terms of diabetic neuropathy, the nerve cells of neuropathy sufferers have been shown to be lower in magnesium than controls. As well, one animal intervention study did find that oral magnesium supplementation to diabetic rats resulted in decreased pain measured by thermal pain thresholds.

The American Diabetes Association recommends assessment of magnesium status in patients at risk for deficiency and supplementation for deficiencies. Since magnesium deficiency may be the most common deficiency in persons with diabetes, and since deficiency may result in progression of diabetic complications, magnesium supplementation is highly recommended. Research suggests that relatively high doses of magnesium for three months, followed by lower daily supplements, are needed to restore and maintain magnesium in people with diabetes.

Good dietary sources include whole grains, leafy green vegetables, legumes, nuts, and fish. Organic sources of these foods have been shown to be as much as 10 times higher in minerals versus conventionally farmed versions. Note also that diets high in saturated fat, sugar, fructose, caffeine, and alcohol may increase magnesium requirements.

Doses of 300 to 600 mg per day of magnesium citrate are appropriate for patients with normal kidney function. Magnesium therapy should only be undertaken with the guidance of a healthcare practitioner familiar with its use.

Carnitine

Carnitine, also known as L-carnitine or acetyl-l-carnitine, is an amino acid-like compound which is synthesized from two amino acids, lysine and methionine, primarily in the liver and kidneys. Carnitine helps in the metabolism of fat in the body because it is responsible for transporting fatty acids into the fat-burning compartment of the cells. Vitamin C is essential for the synthesis of carnitine. It has been shown that during growth, pregnancy or disease there may be a deficiency of carnitine available. For instance, carnitine levels have been shown to be lower in people with diabetic complications than those persons with diabetes without complications. (1) Another study compared L-carnitine and acetyl-l-carnitine levels in the peripheral nerves of people with diabetic peripheral neuropathy, non-diabetic neuropathy, and normal healthy people. Both groups with neuropathy had lower carnitine and acetyl-l-carnitine levels compared to healthy "controls". (2)

What about giving carnitine as a nutritional supplement to persons with diabetes? In a double-blind placebo-controlled trial, 333 subjects with diabetic neuropathy were given acetyl-l-carnitine or placebo for one year. The dose given was 2,000 mg daily taken orally after having been given a 1,000 mg dose by intra-muscular injection for the first 10 days. Pain was reduced by 39 percent in the carnitine group versus eight percent in the placebo. In addition, objective measurements of nerve function also improved, such as nerve conduction velocity. (3)

Another larger study of 1,346 people investigated a 500 mg or 1,000 mg oral acetyl-l-carnitine dose or placebo three times daily for one year. Vibrational sensation was significantly improved in the fingers of both the 1,500 mg per day and the 3,000 mg per day groups, but in the toes only in the 3,000 mg dose. In this particular study, acetyl-l-carnitine appeared to lessen the severity and shorten the duration of neuropathy. (4)

Additional research done on animals and humans has shown that carnitine may benefit persons with diabetes in a number of ways. For instance, improvements in insulin sensitivity and improved glucose metabolism have been noted. In animal studies, reduced damage from free radicals, and reduced sorbitol levels were found in nerve tissue. Carnitine has also been shown to improve nerve myoinositol levels, an important compound that is excreted by the nerves of persons with diabetes. Carnitine has an excellent safety profile, has been shown to improve nerve symptoms in persons with diabetes, potentially has multiple mechanisms of action, and may help regenerate nerve fibers. It is therefore a highly recommended supplement for persons with diabetes. It has also been used for a wide variety of health concerns including heart disease, high cholesterol, Down syndrome, male infertility and hyperthyroidism.

Remarkable Turn Around after 35 Years of Diabetic Damage

Madeline was 56 years old and in very dire straits. A 35-year history of type 1 diabetes had left her with angina, very poor vision, chronic neuropathic pain in both her feet which made it difficult to walk even three steps, and steadily declining kidney function. Objectively, her facial skin tone was very grey, there was a great deal of swelling and blood pooling around her ankles, and her ankle pulses were diminished. She reported that as much as she tried she could not get a chronic fungal skin rash to clear by applying over-the-counter preparations. Having attended the diabetic clinic for the past 35 years, she was aware that managing blood sugar levels is of critical importance. Yet, no matter which insulin regime she experimented with based on the advice of her doctors, she experienced both blood sugar highs and lows on a regular basis. Her blood work confirmed that she was in poor control with a HbA1c level of 9.2% (4.6-6.5). Madeline's triglycerides were also elevated and her HDL was very low, indicating the likelihood of insulin resistance, which would confound

attempts to balance her glucose levels and put her at an extreme-
ly high risk for a heart attack or stroke. An oral hypoglycemic
drug, prescribed by her doctor, had only accelerated her kidney
damage and had to be discontinued. Madeline's mood was very
somber when she stated that she did not believe she would live
very much longer.

Analysis

Madeline's case is typical in many ways for long-term type
1 diabetes sufferers in that she was experiencing the triad of
diabetic complications known as diabetic retinopathy, diabetic
neuropathy and diabetic nephropathy. On top of that she had
developed insulin resistance due to a high carbohydrate diet
combined with inactivity exacerbated by her inability to walk.
Fungal infections are also common in persons with diabetes due
to excess blood sugar levels. As well, diabetics are prone to high
cholesterol levels and increased risk of heart disease and stroke.

Treatment

Madeline began an intensive diet and supplement regime de-
signed to regulate her blood sugar, prevent further damage
and begin repairing existing damage. This included a probiotic
supplement (for the prevention and treatment of fungal infec-
tions), a blood sugar balancing supplement (Glucose Balance Px
–WTSmed) with each meal, a high-potency vitamin/mineral drink
(Cell Nutrition Px –WTSmed), and a diet focused on low-glyce-
mic foods (under 50 on the glycemic scale). A summary of Made-
line's daily nutrient intake is shown in the table below, given as a

percentage of the US recommended daily intakes, to illustrate the typical levels of nutrients needed to reverse this type of advanced chronic disease.

Madeline's Plan

Summary of Daily Nutrient Intake and US FDA RDI:

Chromium	1,166.67 %
Vitamin C	1,666.67 %
B5	5,000 %
B6	5,000 %
B12	16,667.7 %
Selenium	286 %
D3	1,000 %

Madeline also was prescribed specialized nutrients such as benfotiamine (320 mg/day – AOR Inc.) and green tea catechins (100 mg three times per day – Originbiomed Inc.) to help reverse her diabetic complications.

The Results

On the first follow-up visit, one month after beginning her program, both my receptionist and I noticed a major improvement in Madeline's facial tone and demeanor. Although she could only walk six steps pain-free instead of three previously, and although her vision had not improved at all, she did note that her ability to concentrate had improved and she had experienced no nighttime low blood sugar episodes in the last two weeks.

Two months after beginning treatment, Madeline stated that her "life is coming back." Her angina attacks had been reduced from two per week to once a month, her fungal rash was retreating, she was able to walk 15 steps pain-free, and her shoes were fitting better due to reduced ankle swelling. Most remarkably, Madeline was now able to once again enjoy a pastime which she loved dearly – she was able to read! New blood work confirmed her progress with a new HbA1c level of 7.7, triglycerides lower by half and good cholesterol doubled.

Three months after beginning treatment Madeline reported that she had gone one month without any angina pain, had only occasional numbness in her feet with no pain, and was experiencing restored sensations. She was now able to read from eight to 10 hours in a day. Follow-up blood work showed that Madeline had indeed turned the corner with a HbA1c level of 6.7, marginally above the normal range for a healthy non-diabetic. Yet, in all this time, Madeline had made only minor changes to her insulin regime, cutting back on her insulin doses in response to her blood sugars balancing.

References and Bibliography

1. Tamamogullari N, Silig Y, Icagasioglu S, Atalay A. Carnitine deficiency in diabetes mellitus complications. J Diabetes Complications 1999;13:251-3.

2. Scarpini E, Doneda P, Pizzul S, et al. L-carnitine and acetyl-L-carnitine in human nerves from normal and diabetic subjects. J Peripher Nerv Syst 996;1:157-163.

3. De Grandis D, Minardi C. Acetyl-L-carnitine (levacecarnine) in the treatment of diabetic neuropathy: a long-term, randomized, double-blind placebo-controlled study. Drugs R D 2002;3:223.

4. Sima AA, Calvani M, Mehra M, Amato A. Acetyl-L-carnitine improves pain, nerve regeneration, and vibratory perception in patients with chronic diabetic neuropathy: an analysis of two randomized placebo-controlled trials. Diabetes Care 2005;28:89-94.

5. Mingrone G, Greco AV, Capristo E, et al. L-carnitine improves glucose disposal in type 2 diabetic patients. J Am Coll Nutr 1999;18:77-82.

6. Capaldo B, Napoli R, Di Bonito P, et al. Carnitine improves peripheral glucose disposal in non-insulin-dependent diabetic patients. Diabetes Res Clin Pract 1991;14:191-5.

7. Mingrone G. Carnitine in type 2 diabetes. Ann N Y Acad Sci 2004;1033:99-107.

8. Tamamogullari N, Silig Y, Icagasioglu S, Atalay A. Carnitine deficiency in diabetes mellitus complications. J Diabetes Complications 1999;13:251-253.

9. Uzun N, Sarikaya S, Uluduz D, Aydin A. Peripheric and automatic neuropathy in children with type 1 diabetes mellitus: the effect of L-carnitine treatment on the peripheral and autonomic nervous system. Electromyogr Clin Neurophysiol 2005;45:343-351.

10. Lo Giudice P, Careddu A, Magni G, et al. Autonomic neuropathy in streptozotocin diabetic rats: effect of acetyl-L-carnitine. Diabetes Res Clin Pract 2002;56:173-180.

11. Gorio A, Di Giulio AM, Tenconi B, et al. Peptide alterations in autonomic diabetic neuropathy prevented by acetyl-L-carnitine. Int J Clin Pharmacol Res 1992;12:225-230.

12. Lowitt S, Malone JI, Salem AF, et al. Acetyl-L-carnitine corrects the altered peripheral nerve function of experimental diabetes. Metabolism 1995;44:677-680.

13. Stevens MJ, Lattimer SA, Feldman EL, et al. Acetyl-L-carnitine deficiency as a cause of altered nerve myoinositol content, Na, K-ATPase activity, and motor conduction velocity in the streptozotocin-diabetic rat. Metabolism 1996;45:865-872.

14. Hotta N, Koh N, Sakakibara F, et al. Effect of propionyl-L-carnitine on motor nerve conduction, autonomic cardiac function, and nerve blood flow in rats with streptozotocin-induced diabetes: comparison with aldose reductase inhibitor. J Pharmacol Exp Ther 1996;276:49-55.

Chapter 5

Treating Peripheral Neuropathy

Treating Peripheral Neuropathy, Part 1

Introduction

Considering treatment options for this condition have been gross-ly inadequate. There are only a few oral FDA-approved medica-tions—and these are specifically indicated for diabetic peripheral neuropathy. Since approximately 65 percent of all peripheral neuropathy sufferers are not persons with diabetes the fact that over 20 million Americans suffer from peripheral neuropathy, most people with this condition are "left out in the cold," without many treatment options.

Why is there such a discrepancy between the many people with neuropathy and the paltry few treatments available? There is no one single answer, however a number of factors come into play. Everyone has heard the popular real estate expression—

location, location, location. A variation of this holds true for research and development for cures and treatments. What is needed is: research money, research money, research money! Research funding for peripheral neuropathy has been conspicuously absent. Fund raising for more "more popular" diseases outweighs fund raising for peripheral neuropathy. The two medical conditions for which the most money is raised are HIV/AIDS and breast cancer. Fund raising for circulation problems (including heart disease and stroke) comes in a distant third. It is ironic that heart disease is the number one killer of Americans, yet it does not top the list of money raised. Fund raising and research grants for peripheral neuropathy are literally "off the charts" with regard to how little is raised compared to other medical conditions. All causes are important, and Americans are incredibly generous in their donations to research for various medical conditions and diseases. What is needed is a greater public awareness of the great impact that peripheral neuropathy has on the American population. When this occurs, better and more effective treatments will become available.

Another problem facing medical researchers today is the fact that there often is no one common denominator for the different types of neuropathy. For example, a person with diabetes with peripheral neuropathy will often experience symptoms of numbness, burning and tingling of the feet. Likewise, a person with spinal stenosis (narrowing of the spinal column which "pinches" on the spinal cord), will often produce the exact same symptoms. Due to this fact, medical researchers and clinicians face a major challenge. Rather than coming up with one "silver bullet" to treat or cure the condition, they must develop a variety of treatments to address the many types of neuropathy.

The picture is not all doom and gloom. Advancements have been made in finding more effective ways to treat peripheral neuropathy. Much of the credit goes to the Neuropathy Association, a nonprofit organization created to increase public awareness, raise money for research and development and for finding treatments and cures. The Neuropathy Association has 50,000 active members and supporters, with approximately 120 support groups throughout the United States and abroad. At present the Neuropathy Association has several neuropathy centers at major university hospitals across the country, serving patients with neuropathy by providing treatment and conducting research into causes and cures. For more information, contact:

The Neuropathy Association®, Inc.
60 East 42nd Street
Suite 942
New York, New York, 10165
Telephone: (212) 692-0662
Web site: www.neuropathy.org

The "coming of age" of the baby boomer generation is still another reason that the future looks rosier for the development of more effective treatments for peripheral neuropathy. Peripheral neuropathy can strike a person of any age but it is far more likely that a person over 60-years-old will suffer from the condition. Biotechnical and pharmaceutical companies have taken note of this fact. More money is being spent by these companies to expedite research and development for new therapies for neuropathy. EpiCept, a pharmaceutical company, for example, has developed a topical drug for relief from pain caused by peripheral neuropathies. EpiCept™ NP-1 is a patented formulation which is presently in phase IIb clinical trials with the FDA. Further trials are expected in the ensuing months.

Treating peripheral neuropathy usually requires a combination of medications and therapies to help relieve the discomfort of pain, burning, numbness and tingling. The remainder of this chapter will address the various treatments that are available, including conventional and some "out-of the-box" approaches as well.

Treating Peripheral Neuropathy, Part 2
Prescription Pharmaceuticals

Gabapentin

Brand names: Neurontin® Gabarone®

About gabapentin

Gabapentin is an oral medication approved by the FDA for the treatment of seizures for patients who have epilepsy. Gabapentin is classified as an anticonvulsant medication. It is also indicated to help relieve nerve pain associated with shingles (also called postherpetic neuralgia). While this medication is one of the most prescribed, it was not developed as a primary treatment for any type of peripheral neuropathy. Since its introduction on market in 1994, gabapentin has been used for a variety of chronic painful conditions including diabetic peripheral neuropathy. It is also used to help relieve discomfort from "hot flashes" in menopausal women. The mechanism of action of how gabapentin relieves nerve pain is not exactly known. Gabapentin is not intended to reverse nerve damage.

Side effects can include:

- Allergic reaction (including hives, difficulty breathing, swelling of your face, lips, tongue, or throat).
- Drowsiness
- Dizziness
- Headache
- Weakness
- Double or blurred vision
- Nausea
- Vomiting
- Heartburn
- Dry mouth
- Weight gain
- Swelling of the hands, feet and legs
- Fever
- Memory problems
- Anxiety
- Constipation
- Joint pain
- Tremors
- Rash
- Itching
- Seizures

Other adverse reactions caused interactions with other medications including prescription and over-the-counter medications (check with your primary care physician before taking gabapentin).

Dosage

A specific protocol and dosage have not been established for gabapentin. Dosages for the condition range from 200 mg to 1,800 mg daily. Higher daily dosages have been prescribed but should be taken with caution.

Special consideration

If gabapentin is reduced or discontinued, it should be tapered slowly, under the supervision of a physician.

Pregabalin

Brand Name: Lyrica®

About Lyrica

Lyrica is an oral medication that is chemically related to Neurontin®. It has been approved by the FDA only for the management of pain from diabetic neuropathy. It also has been approved by the FDA for other conditions including pain from shingles (postherpetic neuralgia), fibromyalgia and as adjunctive therapy (meaning working in combination with other medications) for adults with partial onset seizures. Lyrica has not been approved by the FDA for the treatment of other kinds of peripheral neuropathy. Lyrica binds voltage-dependent calcium channels in the central nervous system—meaning that it works by attaching to part of an over-firing nerve cell. In theory this is thought to reduce pain signals in patients with diabetic peripheral neuropathy. It should be noted that the exact mechanism of how Lyrica works to relieve diabetic nerve pain is not entirely known.

As with Neurontin, caution should be used before driving a car since Lyrica can adversely affect your alertness and vision. Do not drink alcohol when taking Lyrica. Lyrica will not reverse the condition of damaged nerves.

Side effects can include:

- Allergic reaction (difficulty breathing, swelling of your face, lips, tongue, or throat)
- Dizziness
- Muscle pain
- Muscle weakness or tenderness
- Easy bruising or bleeding
- Swelling in your hands or feet
- Anxiety
- Loss of balance
- Problems with memory or concentration
- Dry mouth
- Skin rash or itching
- Constipation
- Increased appetite and weight gain

- Drowsiness

- Blurred vision

- Reduced platelet count

- Muscle injury from increased blood levels of a chemical called creatine kinase

Other adverse reactions caused interactions with other medications including prescription and over-the-counter medications. (check with your primary care physician before taking Lyrica)

Dosage

The starting dose for diabetic peripheral neuropathy is 50 mg three times a day or 75 mg twice a day. The maximum recommended dose is 300 mg a day.

Special considerations

If Lyrica is reduced or discontinued, it should be tapered slowly, under the supervision of a physician.

Duloxetine

Brand name: Cymbalta®

About Cymbalta

Cymbalta is an antidepressant medication. It is used to treat major depressive disorders and general anxiety disorder. It is in the category of antidepressants called selective serotonin and norepinephrine reuptake inhibitors—SSNRI's. Cymbalta has also been approved by the FDA to manage pain associated with diabetic peripheral neuropathy.

Cymbalta, and other SSNRI medications, increase the amounts of serotonin and norepinephrine in the brain of patients lacking in these chemicals. Adequate amounts of serotonin and norepinephrine help maintain emotional balance. Studies have shown that Cymbalta may reduce pain signals to the brain. However, the exact mechanism of how Cymbalta works is not entirely known.

Cymbalta will not reverse damage but may reduce pain caused by diabetic peripheral neuropathy. Since Cymbalta can cause drowsiness and dizziness, caution should be used when driving a car. Avoid drinking alcohol when taking Cymbalta.

Side effects include:

- Nausea
- Constipation
- Diarrhea

- Dry mouth
- Insomnia
- Weight changes
- Sweating
- Tremors
- Urinary difficulties
- Vomiting
- Sexual difficulties
- Jaundice
- Fatigue
- Allergic reaction including rash, hives or difficulty breathing

Special considerations

Do not take Cymbalta together with other MAO (monoamine oxidase inhibitors are a class of powerful antidepressant medications) drugs including Marplan®, Parnate®, Nardil®, Azilect® or Eldepryl®. Do not use Cymbalta with thioridazine (Mellaril®). Serious or sometimes fatal reactions can occur when these medications are taken with Cymbalta.

Dosage

The recommended dosage for diabetic peripheral neuropathy is 60 mg once a day.

Tricyclic Antidepressants (TCA's)

These medications were used for treating peripheral neuropathy although they have not been approved by the FDA specifically for pain management.

Brand names:

Tofranil® (imipramine)

Elavil® (amitriptyline)

Pamelor® (nortriptyline)

Norpramin® (desipramine)

Sinequan® (doxepin)

About tricyclic antidepressants (TCA)

Certain brain chemicals called neurotransmitters (including serotonin, norepinephrine and dopamine) are associated with depression. Like the medication Cymbalta, these antidepressants work by inhibiting the uptake of these neurotransmitters. Tricyclics are also known to be effective in treating certain chronic painful conditions including peripheral neuropathy, shingles, migraines and fibromyalgia.

The exact mechanism of how tricyclics work to reduce pain (called an analgesic effect) is not fully understood. It is postulated that TCA work by regulating amounts of neurotransmitters in our system. This action may help block and reduce pain signals.

The primary use of tricyclic antidepressants remains as a treatment for depression. Like all other medications mentioned in this chapter, TCA will not reverse nerve damage but may be helpful in reducing pain, burning and tingling associated with peripheral neuropathy.

Side effects

Since tricyclic antidepressants are less selective about which cells they affect, they can have more side effects than other antidepressants. Side effects include:

- Drowsiness
- Blurred vision
- Memory difficulties
- Weakness
- Nausea
- Vomiting
- Dizziness
- Low blood pressure
- Impaired sexual function
- Constipation
- Difficulty urinating
- Weight gain
- Irregular heart rate
- Sweating
- Sensitivity to light
- Allergic reactions including rash, hives or difficulty breathing

Special considerations

Caution should be used when taking other medications as you may experience adverse or even fatal reactions. These include antipsychotics such as Clonidine, MAO inhibitors like Marplan®, Parnate®, Nardil®, Azilect® or Eldepryl® and when used in combination with other tricyclics.

Other adverse reactions may occur with different classes of medications such as:

- Medication for asthma
- Cimetidine (Tagamet®) for relief of heartburn
- Medications for colds, hay fever or allergies
- Heart medication (Isuprel®)
- Gastrointestinal medications (Reglan®)
- Medication for attention-deficit/hyperactivity disorder (Cylert®)
- Some antihypertensive medications (Aldomet®, Demser® and Hylorel®)
- Antihistamine agents (Phenergan®)
- Radioopaque agents (Metrizamide)

Drinking alcohol should be avoided when taking tricyclic antidepressants.

Other Pain Medications

The medications just discussed are the "standards" for treating peripheral neuropathy and are usually the first ones prescribed by the health care professional. Often times these medications are not effective in relieving the discomfort associated with peripheral neuropathy. Some people simply cannot tolerate the side effects of these drugs. In such instances your physician may elect to use other analgesic medications. There are literally hundreds of over-the-counter and prescription medications. The medication chosen by your doctor will depend on a number of factors including the severity of symptoms, consideration of your over all general health and medications that you are presently taking for existing medical problems. It is beyond the scope of this book to discuss pain medications in detail however a general overview will be presented.

Over-the-counter Medications

Acetaminophen (Tylenol®) is a "milder" pain medication with generally fewer side effects than aspirin or nonsteroidal anti-inflammatory medications (referred to as NSAID). People with liver disease should avoid taking this medication.

Aspirin is the "gold standard" for pain medication. Aspirin does have a number of side effects, including gastrointestinal problems such as nausea, vomiting, diarrhea and constipation. Aspirin may cause stomach ulcers if taken over a prolonged period of time. This pain-relieving medication may also affect the blood-clotting mechanism of the body, causing delay in clotting times.

Other pain medications fall in the category of non-steroidal anti-inflammatory medication. Some of the more common drugs in this class include Aleve®, Motrin® and Advil®). Like aspirin, NSAID's can cause gastrointestinal upset (nausea, vomiting, diarrhea or constipation), along with stomach ulcers, delayed clotting times, renal (kidney) and liver problems.

Prescription Pain Medications

These medications are generally used for people who have higher levels of symptoms, including more severe pain, tingling and burning. These "stronger" analgesics may be associated with more side effects. Medications in this category are called opioids and include codeine (including Tylenol® with Codeine and Vicodin®), Darvon®, Darvocet-N®, and oxycodone (OxyContin®, Percocet® and Percodan®). The most potent opioids are morphine and methadone and should only be used in the most extreme cases.

Side Effects

Each of the medications listed above have their own side effects and caution must be used when they are taken, particularly over longer periods of time. Many of the opioids have certain side effects in common which include:

- Long-term use can lead to physical dependence, tolerance, addiction and abuse

- Respiratory depression which can affect breathing capacity. This is one of the most serious adverse reactions associated with opioid use

- Nausea and vomiting

- Drowsiness

- Constipation—this develops in over 95 percent of patients taking opioids over a prolonged period of time

- Dry mouth

- Confusion

- Dizziness

- Headache

- Urinary retention

- Heartbeat irregularities including bradycardia (slowing of heart rate) or tachycardia (speeding up of the heart rate)

- "Itching"—urticaria

- Orthostatic hypotention which is a sudden drop in blood pressure when a person assumes a standing position. This condition can cause dizziness or fainting

Special Considerations

All pain medications may interact adversely with other prescription and non-prescription medications that you are taking, including certain vitamins and nutritional supplements. It is imperative that you inform your health care professional of all medications that you are presently taking before any pain medication is prescribed. Drinking alcohol should be avoided when taking any pain medication.

When taking oral medications for peripheral neuropathy you should take an active role in helping your physician decide if any of these drugs are right for you. In other words: communication with your doctor is vitally important. Before taking any medications it is helpful to articulate the type of pain or discomfort you are experiencing. Rating pain, burning, tingling and other symptoms causing discomfort on a scale of zero to 10 (0 being no pain and 10 being unbearable pain) can be most helpful in choosing an appropriate medication.

It is also very important to have realistic expectations. Keep in mind that in most instances peripheral neuropathy is not curable. The goal when using oral medications is to reduce discomfort and thus improve quality of life. It is not realistic to think that one medication will totally eliminate all symptoms of peripheral neuropathy.

Be your own advocate when deciding to take oral medications. If you do not think a medication is helping to control your neuropathy symptoms, inform your doctor of this fact. We often hear patients tell us at the Foot Pain Center that they are taking high doses of medications such as over 2,000 mg of gabapentin on a daily basis. When questioned if the medication is helping, a common response is "I'm not sure. I still have a lot of discomfort but I continue to take it because my doctor prescribed it." Other people relate that they experience uncomfortable side effects including drowsiness, weight gain and a host of other complications, yet they try to "work through it" and continue to take the medication.

A word of caution: never discontinue taking a medication without telling your physician first. Dosages for medications such as Neurontin and Lyrica should be reduced gradually.

Oral medications may not be right for you, and in many instances it is a "trial and error" process to make that determination. Fortunately, other treatment methods have been developed which may be more effective and have fewer side effects. These treatments will be discussed in the next chapter.

Treating Peripheral Neuropathy, Part 3
Therapy Treatments—Laser, Infrared and More

Traditionally the medical community has treated peripheral neuropathy in a "hands-off" manner, meaning that in most instances, the affected areas on the feet and hands are actually never touched. As noted in the previous chapters, the primary approach has always been by the use medications, either oral or topical. Some of the greatest advancements in the treatment of peripheral neuropathy have been by the utilization of "hands-on" therapy treatments. Keep in mind in most instances no therapy treatment, no matter how sophisticated, will not "cure" the condition and will not reverse nerve damage. The purpose of treatment is to help reduce the discomfort caused by peripheral neuropathy. At The Foot Pain Center, our approach is to use various therapies treatments as a way to manage neuropathic pain. Many of these treatments are performed in the office and some are available for home use. Both types will be discussed in this chapter.

Infrared Therapy

What is Infrared Therapy

Many treatments that are used for neuropathic pain were developed for other medical conditions. Many infrared therapy units have been devised to specifically treat pain, numbness and burning. A little physics lesson first. The electromagnetic spectrum consists of energy particles (measured in units called nanometers) of different wavelengths. The longest wavelengths are radio waves and shortest are x-rays (gamma rays). In the middle of this energy spectrum are visible light waves. Visible light ranges from the shortest—violet light which is 400 nanometers, to the longest—red light which is 700 nanometers. Infrared light has a length of 890 nanometers which is outside the spectrum of visible light. Infrared light therapy is also known as monochromatic infrared photo energy.

How Does Infrared Therapy Work?

Infrared therapy in the reduction of neuropathic pain has been the subject of many extensive studies. How infrared therapy works to help reduce pain, numbness, burning and tingling is not entirely clear. It is postulated that light energy at this specific wavelength helps increase local circulation to nerves and other tissue. The vasodilatation effect (increasing circulation to the area) seems to have a direct effect on reducing pain and numbness. Infrared light is also thought to stimulate release of the chemical, nitric oxide. Many studies have shown that this chemical plays an important role in maintaining healthy circulation. Nitric oxide is also used by the body for neurotransmission of certain chemicals which are essential for proper nerve conduction.

How is Infrared Therapy Administered?

Since most symptoms of peripheral neuropathy are manifested in the lower extremities many infrared devices are made in the shape of a boot to conform to the feet and legs. Treatments are usually scheduled two or three times a week, for a period of four to six weeks, with each treatment lasting from 30 to 50 minutes. After that, treatments can be administered on "as needed basis." Physicians, podiatrists and physical therapists, especially those who see many neuropathy patients, will often have professional infrared units in their offices.

Are Infrared Units Available for Home Use?

Yes. Caution is advised before purchasing a home infrared unit since they can be costly. Higher quality units can range from $1,000 to $2,500. It is strongly suggested that you "do your homework" before making a purchase of this magnitude. Make sure that the manufacturer's claims are substantiated by appropriate documented studies. It is advisable that the unit you are considering purchasing is FDA cleared. Since infrared treatments do not involve the use of medication, such devices do not have to be FDA approved. Certain standards must be met to receive FDA clearance. FDA clearance also means that the particular manufacturer is registered and on record with this agency. Another important tip, if you intend to purchase a unit, is to make sure that the company you are purchasing from has a 30-day money-back guarantee if you are not satisfied with the results.

Advantages and Disadvantages of Infrared Therapy

Although many studies have shown that infrared therapy can help reduce neuropathic pain, the results are not always conclusive or consistent. A major advantage of infrared therapy is that it is entirely drug-free with very few side effects. A contraindication to the use of infrared therapy is pregnancy. Also infrared therapy should not be used over areas of active cancer such as skin cancers like malignant melanoma. At The Foot Pain Center we have found that infrared therapy is often more effective when used in conjunction with other therapies and medications. Overall infrared is safe, convenient to use and can be effective in certain cases.

Laser Therapy

There are many types of medical lasers used to treat of variety of conditions. The YAG laser, for example, is used to treat eye problems such as cataracts. The kind used for treating neuropathic pain is called low-level laser light therapy. Like infrared, low-level laser therapy uses light in the spectrum of red and near infrared light. Low-level lasers supply energy to the body in the form of non-thermal (energy without heat) photons of light. This type of laser can penetrate deeper into the tissues of the body because of its unique properties. Laser light is coherent, monochromatic and polarized. This means that the light travels in a straight line, contains just a single wavelength of energy and the beam is concentrated to a defined location. This is exactly opposite of the light seen in a rainbow. A rainbow is in the shape of an arc (not a straight line), is made up of many colors in the light spectrum and is not concentrated to one spot.

Low-level laser units are available in different strengths of power, measured in milliwatts. Lasers which can deliver more milliwatts of power can speed up the treatment process and also can penetrate deeper into the affected nerves. The laser energy is administered by a wand or probe applied directly to the skin. In general, laser was developed for many conditions but not specifically for the treatment of peripheral neuropathy. The physiological effects of low-level laser include:

- Improved cell metabolism through bio-stimulation
- Improved circulation and vasodilatation
- Analgesic effect (pain relief)
- Anti-inflammatory (reduced swelling)
- Stimulation of wound healing

As a result of these beneficial effects, low-level laser therapy definitely has a place in the treatment of peripheral neuropathy. This type of laser treatment can help relieve acute and chronic pain, including neuropathic pain. It has been shown to stimulate proper nerve function. Like its cousin infrared therapy, it is unlikely that laser will reverse nerve damage. The vasodilatation effect of low-level also helps to reduce pain, tingling and numbness.

How is Laser Administered?

The laser energy is administered by a wand or a probe which is applied directly to the skin. The amount of energy delivered by laser is measured in joules. Guidelines for treatment of specific conditions have been established. For example, in treating neuropathic pain, a total of 100-200 joules per treatment is the recommended dosage of energy. Depending on the power output of the laser unit (with a higher output unit requiring less time) average treatment times range from 30 seconds to two minutes per foot.

Are Laser Units Available for Home Use?

For the most part, no.

The FDA has developed a classification system which rates laser safety. The system ranges from Class I lasers which are the safest to Class IV lasers which can cause the most damage, especially to the eyes. Class I and II lasers will not damage the eyes. Laser light emitted in these classes can be purchased by anyone and are really not used for medical conditions. Included in this class are laser pointers. Be wary of anyone making claims that lasers in these categories can be used for beneficial medical purposes. These lasers are safe but barely emit enough laser energy to penetrate through the skin.

Lasers included in Class III and IV can cause permanent eye damage and protective eyewear must always be worn when they are being used. These low-level laser devices should only be used by physicians, podiatrists and chiropractors who have had training in administering laser therapy. These are the most effective lasers for treating peripheral neuropathy and other conditions. They are the most powerful and can penetrate deepest into bodily tissue. Lasers in classes II and IV cannot be purchased by non-medical personnel.

Advantages and Disadvantages of Low-Level Laser Therapy

Low-level laser is non-invasive and drug-free. It is gaining popularity as a definitive treatment for chronic painful conditions. Its use for treating neuropathic pain is a relatively new application and is proving to be quite effective. A range of treatments doses (in joules) is recommended, but no exact protocol has been established. It takes some trial and error to determine the most effective dose of laser energy. Treatment times are short—less than two minutes making it quite convenient. A disadvantage is the fact that not many medical facilities have low-level laser units, especially for the treatment of neuropathy. Lasers, specifically Class III and IV, carry a risk of eye damage. Protective goggles should always be worn and therapy should be performed by health care professionals who have had experience and training in administering low level laser.

Electric-Medical Therapy

Electric-medical therapy, also known has electrical stimulation, is the use of various devices that generate a low voltage current for the purpose of pain control, including neuropathic pain. Electrical stimulation has been used by the medical community for the past 40 years. This type of therapy stimulates nerves and blocks pain signals before they can be received by the brain.

Types of Electric-Medical Therapy

TENS Therapy

The most commonly used device is Transcutaneous Nerve Stimulation, referred to as TENS therapy. A TENS unit is a compact portable device about the size of a cell phone. The unit is operated by a battery and emits an electric current. The low voltage current then passes from the unit via thin wires to electrodes, which are pads that adhere to the skin. Once placed on the skin in the areas of pain, the pads conduct the current to the level of the nerve fibers, approximately one or two inches deep. This current "short-circuits" pain messages from the brain. This process is helpful in breaking the pain cycle. TENS therapy is used to treat any acute and chronic painful condition, including bursitis, headaches, back pain and a host of other medical problems. TENS therapy is an effective modality in treating neuropathic pain as it is targeted to penetrate to the level of nerve fibers.

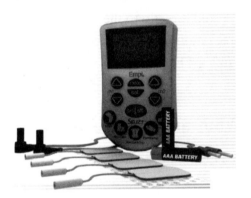

Fig. 5: TENS Device

Availability for Home Use

Yes. TENS was designed to be a self-administered, home therapy treatment. Being small and lightweight, the TENS device can fit on a belt or placed in a small pocket. The user can choose from a variety of setting and programs. The person using the device can set the length of treatment and the amount of electrical current going in to the electrodes. Treatment times can vary from 30 minutes to many hours. There are also many programs to choose from, including continual output of electrical current to a pause or delay in output. It is often a personal choice depending on a person's comfort level and tolerance to the treatment.

Are TENS Units Available by Prescription?

Yes and no. Many health care professional will prescribe a TENS unit as an adjunct to other medications and therapies being used to treat your condition. Some insurance companies (you need to check your policy) may provide a TENS device if certain criteria are met. A search on the Internet reveals that many devices are sold directly to the consumer without a prescription. Certain precautions apply and you should check with your doctor before using a TENS unit.

What are the Precautions?

A TENS unit should not be used by anyone who has a pacemaker, defibrillator or during pregnancy. People with neck and head pain should be monitored by a health care professional on proper placement of the electrodes. Caution should be used when driving while wearing a TENS unit as the therapy may cause a distraction.

Advantages and Disadvantages of TENS Therapy

TENS therapy is drug free and is safe as long as the precautions are followed. The big plus of TENS therapy is that it is mobile and designed for home use. It can be applied at any time during the day or evening when you are experiencing pain. A disadvantage is that it may be difficult to decide which unit to purchase since there are so many devices available to the consumer. Do some research before purchasing a unit or ask your physician. TENS therapy may or may not be effective in treating neuropathic pain. Since it is safe, readily available and drug free, it is probably worth a try.

Interferential Electrical Stimulation

Interferential electrical stimulation is similar to TENS therapy with one major difference: The electrical stimulation is delivered to affected area by "crossing" the wires. This allows the current to be delivered deeper into the tissue than an ordinary TENS unit. The electrical frequencies generated by interferential current interfere with the transmission of pain messages at the spinal cord level. The same precautions as noted for TENS apply to interferential therapy. Interferential is drug free and is as safe as TENS therapy. Interferential therapy is often administered by physicians or therapists in their offices using professional units. Home units are also available that can be used in a TENS or interferential mode.

Ionotophoresis

Ionotophoresis is a physical therapy treatment which is used to treat chronic painful conditions. It is a technique whereby prescription medications can be passed through the skin by electrical current without the need for injections. Physical therapists often use ionotophoresis to treat tendonitis and soft tissue injuries. The Foot Pain Center and other facilities are now using this technique to treat pain, burning and tingling often associated with peripheral neuropathy.

Ionotophoresis works as follows: The treating physician will select a specific medication, or combination of medications, for the ionotophoresis treatment. Common medications used for peripheral neuropathy include gabapentin, ketamine and baclofen. A specialized pharmacist (called a compound pharmacist) will prepare a liquid solution containing these medications. The solution is applied to an electrical pad and the medication passes through the skin using a mild, low-level electrical current.

More About Ionotophoresis

Ionotophoresis has been used by health care professionals for the treatment of a variety of chronic painful conditions. Its application for use in treating peripheral neuropathy is relatively new. At The Foot Pain Center, ionotophoresis has been used on over 500 patients with very encouraging results. Many patients have reported reduction of pain, burning and tingling following a series of treatments using ionotophoresis.

Ionotophoresis has advantages over the use of oral and topical medications. As noted in previous chapters, oral medications such as gabapentin have many side effects. Topical treatments such as analgesic creams, lotions and gels often have difficulty passing through the thick and toughened skin on the sole of the foot. Medications using ionotophoresis can pass easily through the skin barrier using a small electric current. The amount of medication that actually gets into the blood stream is very minimal, thus reducing side effects. Contraindications to ionotophoresis include allergy to any of the medication being used. Also patients with a pacemaker or defibrillator cannot use this therapy because of the presence of an electrical current.

Massage Therapy

Massage therapy dates back to the ancient civilizations of Egypt, Greece and Rome. The technical definition of massage is manipulation by hand, or with an instrument, to any body part using a degree of pressure. Targeted body structures include muscles, tendons, nerves, ligaments, skin, joints or lymphatic vessels. There are over 70 documented types of massage therapies.

Benefits of Massage

Both formal medical studies and subjective input from patients indicate an overwhelming positive response and with many associated benefits of massage. Benefits include:

- Pain relief
- Improved circulation
- Relaxation
- Easing of tension and stiffness
- Promoting the healing of soft tissue injuries

Contraindications of Massage

Massage should not be used in an area were a deep blood clot is suspected. A person who experiences swelling or a sharp or dull pain in the thigh or calf should seek medical attention immediately.

Any person who has had a DVT (deep thrombophlebitis) should check with their physician before undergoing massage therapy.

Massage therapy should not be used on an area where an acute injury such as a fracture is suspected.

Many massage therapies are tailored for pregnant women and care should be taken to avoid excessive pressure on the uterine area.

More about Massage Therapy

At The Foot Pain Center, massage therapy is used regularly and has been found to be one of the effective "hands on" treatments for peripheral neuropathy. As previously discussed, massage facilitates increasing local circulation to an area, including damaged nerves. Increased blood flow to damaged nerves helps reduce pain, tingling and burning in the affected area. Massage therapy can temporarily reduce the "feeling of numbness" associated with peripheral neuropathy.

Temporary is the key word. Despite its many benefits, massage therapy will not permanently reverse nerve damage. It is an excellent adjunctive treatment when used in conjunction with oral, topical or other forms of therapy for neuropathic pain.

Another advantage of massage therapy is that it is a great stress-reducer. Peripheral neuropathy sufferers have to continually cope with the many adverse effects of the condition including severe discomfort and loss of balance. These chronic symptoms invariably produce both physical and emotional stress. Periodic massage therapy can help control and lessen stress created by this condition.

A Final Word on Massage Therapy

Massage therapy is performed by a massage therapist, physician, osteopath, chiropractor, or physical therapist. Home massage units are available to patients who would like to self-treat on a daily, or as-needed, basis. There are many excellent home units for sale to the public. The Foot Pain Center uses a foot massager and a separate body massager for in-office treatments by a company called Medi-Rub® Corporation. These same professional units are available for purchase for home use.

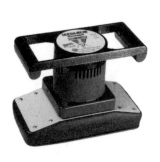
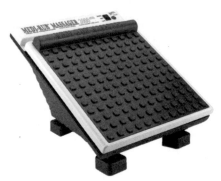

Fig. 6: Medi-Rub® foot massager

Fig. 7: Medi-Rub® body massager

Chapter 6

Topical Treatments for PN

Introduction

The approach of using topical formulations for peripheral neuropathy appeals to many people. For one thing, most people don't like to take pills. Therefore, any pain medication in the form of a lotion, cream, patch or ointment which can be applied topically, directly to the area of discomfort, is of great interest to many people. Topical medications also tend to have far fewer or less severe side effects than their oral cousins. One reason for this is that very little of the drug is absorbed into the circulatory system. To appreciate the difference between oral and topical medications it helps to understand the types of nervous systems in the body.

The nerves which make up the human body are divided into two groups: those of the central nervous system, which consists of the brain and spinal cord, and those of the peripheral nervous system, which consists of all the rest of the nerves in the body, such as those found in the arms and legs. The name "peripheral neuropathy" of course refers to the fact that the problem nerves in this condition are found in the peripheral nervous system. The great advantage of topical treatments for PN is that a topical treatment can target the specific area where the pain originates, such as the feet, with very little or no effect on the brain. In other words, since there is very little drug circulating in the body, there is much less chance that the medication will affect the other nervous system (i.e., the central nervous system) with unwanted side effects.

This avoids the most common side effects associated with current oral medications for PN, such as fatigue, weight gain and mood disturbances, which are due to the undesirable effect of the drug on the brain. In fact, the current crop of oral drugs approved for treating PN were actually designed primarily for another purpose, either as anti-seizure medications or antidepressants. Both these types of medications target the brain specifically and intentionally. This makes them effective for preventing seizures and treating depression, but not particularly suited to the treatment of pain in the toes.

Unwanted drug effects can also be caused by the strain put on the organs of detoxification, such as the liver and kidneys. It is the job of these organs to clear drugs and toxins from the body. These organs can become damaged by the extra load put on them by a drug over a long period of time or in some cases even a short time, if the medication is difficult to detoxify, the person is taking a cocktail of medications and/or recreational drugs, or the person already has compromised organ function. Drugs are also notorious for interacting with other drugs or even with herbal medicines and foods, resulting in even more unwanted effects. Both these tendencies are minimized by the use of topical formulations. With topical formulations, so little is absorbed into the circulation there is very little extra load placed on the organs of detoxification, and very little chance of unwanted interactions with other drugs or foods. Many people have found that topical treatments for neuropathic pain relief are the best choice among medications.

Types of Topical Medications for PN

- Ointments contain little if any water and generally feel greasy. Drugs in ointments are often more potent than in creams.

- Lotions originally were suspensions of powdered material (e.g., calamine) in a water or alcohol base; most modern lotions (e.g., some corticosteroids) are water-based emulsions. They are convenient to apply and often feel cooling to the skin.

- Solutions are homogenous mixtures of two or more substances. Solutions are drying and easy to apply. The most commonly used bases are ethyl alcohol, propylene glycol, polyethylene glycol and water.

- Patches are topical drug delivery systems which contain a reservoir of medication in the middle and a surrounding adhesive which attaches the patch to the skin.

Over-the-Counter Topical Treatments

Neuragen®

Neuragen is a natural, topical over-the-counter product which was designed to relieve neuropathic pain. In clinical trials to date, Neuragen, when applied topically, has been shown to be effective in a group of "all-cause" neuropathy sufferers. "All cause" refers to a group with painful neuropathy due to various conditions such as diabetic peripheral neuropathy, chemo-induced neuropathy, HIV neuropathy, and idiopathic (unknown cause) neuropathy, etc. Forty subjects with all cause neuropathic pain in the feet were treated in a double blind placebo controlled trial by independent researchers at Louisiana State University. The graph below represents the average pain level for all participants before treatment (time=0) and for up to nine hours after treatment with either Neuragen (drops) or placebo (triangles). Pain relief with Neuragen was statistically significant over placebo and for up to eight hours in duration.

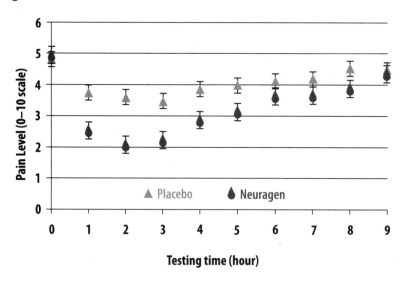

Fig. 8: Neuragen Trial Over Nine Hours

Users of Neuragen typically report pain relief within fifteen minutes that lasts for two to eight hours after only a few drops are applied topically. Overall, approximately 80% of subjects reported some pain relief, with 63% of subjects receiving Neuragen benefitting from a 50% or greater reduction in pain (vs. only 15% in the placebo group). As with many topical approaches, there is very little concern about side effects or drug interactions.

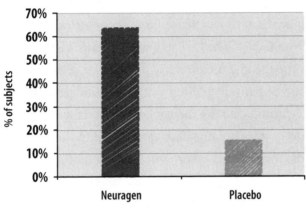

Fig. 9: Neuragen Pain Relief

Capsaicin

Capsaicin is a medication derived from cayenne peppers. Capsaicin is the chemical within the peppers responsible for the burning sensation that people get when cayenne comes in contact with the skin, mucous membranes, or, as most chefs have had the misfortune to discover, when rubbed in the eye. The potency of peppers has long been appreciated. The Mayans burned chili peppers to make stinging smoke screens and flung pepper-filled gourds at their enemies. The Japanese even found a way to keep crop-eating monkeys out of farmers' fields by shooting chili powder into the air, irritating the eyes and noses of the primates.

More recently, pepper has been used in sprays to fend off dogs, bears, would-be assailants, and used by police to contain unruly protestors.

Capsaicin is not only used to treat neuropathy but may also provide pain relief from back problems, bursitis, postherpetic neuralgia, arthritis, joint pain, and pruritus (itching). For the treatment of neuropathic pain, capsaicin is typically delivered in the form of a cream, such as Zostrix®, which is 0.025% capsaicin. Capsaicin is not an anesthetic but acts to relieve pain by causing nerve cells to release large amounts of a chemical called "substance P." The "P" stands for "Pain." Substance P is believed to be the chemical released by nerve cells which causes the sensation of pain. Depletion of this peptide neurotransmitter from nerve endings, so the theory goes, means that pain impulses cannot be as readily created and transmitted to the brain. In other words, the nerve is "worn out" and cannot muster another pain signal. The problem is that it may take some time to "wear out" the nerve's supply of substance P. An initial burning sensation is usually experienced during the first several days, and this increase in pain above and beyond the pain they already have deters many from using capsaicin products. Capsaicin is generally applied three to four times daily to the affected area. Most practitioners agree that if a patient is not willing to use a capsaicin product at least three times a day for an extended period, the patient should not bother with this therapy. For those wishing to try capsaicin, it is wise to start with a very small area of skin to check one's ability to tolerate this approach. When using the cream, lotion or gel, apply a thin layer of medication to the areas of maximum pain or discomfort using a cotton swab or wearing Latex gloves. Care must be taken to avoid touching capsaicin with your hands. An additional note of caution is warranted with this approach: Do not apply to the eyes, mouth, nostrils or genitals. Do not apply to injured or irritated skin. Since capsaicin produces the sensation of heat, it is strongly recommended to avoid activities which may heat up the area where the capsaicin has been applied. Such activities would include bathing in warm water, sun bathing or strenuous activities. If applied to the feet, wait at least 30 minutes before putting on socks or shoes.

There are now even higher-potency versions of capsaicin available, but these seem to be intolerable to almost everyone without a local anesthetic first injected at the site of the cream application to lessen the intense burning sensation. Also of interest is that a number of people with peripheral neuropathy have noted improvements by taking cayenne pepper capsules orally as opposed to topical use.

Ben-Gay®

Ben-Gay is a topical pain reliever based on methyl salicylate (a similar ingredient to aspirin) combined with menthol, an essential oil found in many plants including mint. Although promoted mainly for muscle and joint pain, it sometimes helps with the tingling and burning of neuropathy. Ben-Gay was developed in the late 1800s by Dr. Bengue, a French pharmacist, and is available as a topical cream and patch.

Prescription Topical Treatments

Lidocaine

Lidocaine is an anesthetic which blocks sodium channels, thereby inhibiting the transmission of pain impulses along neurons. Lidocaine patches are approved by the FDA for the treatment of postherpetic neuralgia, a type of chronic neuropathic pain caused by the herpes zoster (shingles) infection. Other studies have shown that lidocaine may also be effective for other types of neuropathies, such as diabetic peripheral neuropathy and HIV neuropathy. Lidoderm® is a patch containing 5% lidocaine. Lidocaine creams are also available. One common side effect of lidocaine is loss of sensation (numbness) over the area of application. Mexitil® is an oral drug with a similar structure to lidocaine, which has benefited some people with peripheral neuropathy, especially the burning component of the pain. However, Mexitil also has effects on heart rate and rhythm, and therefore must be used with caution as it may cause palpitations and/or irregular heart rhythm (arrhythmia).

Precautions When Using the Lidoderm Patch

Lidocaine, which is structurally similar to Novocaine®, is most often used as a local anesthetic to "numb" a particular area on the body. Lidoderm is usually dispensed in a carton containing 30 patches. When used in treating peripheral neuropathy pain, a patch is applied directly over the area of discomfort. A maximum of three patches can be used daily. The patch can remain in place for twelve hours and then must be removed.

The patch is most often well tolerated but in rare instances side effects can occur which may include:

- Allergic reaction: People who have a known reaction to any to the "caines"—such as lidocaine (Xylocaine®), mepivacaine (Carbocaine®), bupivacaine (Marcaine®) and all others— should not use this product. A rare but severe allergic or anaphylactoid reaction may occur.

- Irritation of the skin at the site of application: Some people may develop skin irritation including rash, blisters, depigmentation (loss of skin color), and localized swelling.

- Drug interactions: The Lidoderm patch should be used with caution in patients receiving Class I antiarryhthmic drugs (medication to control an irregular heart beat).

- Other adverse reactions: May include dizziness, a lightheaded feeling, metallic taste or blurred vision.

Advantages/disadvantages of the Lidoderm Patch

The patch is usually well tolerated with minimal side effects. Since it can be applied to an area of discomfort for up to 12 hours, it can have a longer-lasting, time-released effect. The Lidoderm patch is not the most effective agent in treating neuropathic pain. A disadvantage of the patch is that as an analgesic medication, it may exacerbate the feeling of numbness which many peripheral neuropathy sufferers already experience. The Lidoderm patch was not intended to treat peripheral neuropathy, so any benefits derived from this product, such as relief from tingling and burning, can be considered a bonus.

Compounded Preparations

Compound pharmaceuticals are used by dermatologists, pediatricians, neurologists, podiatrists and sports medicine specialists. There is no one standard formulation for reducing pain and discomfort associated with peripheral neuropathy. Physicians will often use their best judgment and experience in formulating compounded topical medications for neuropathic pain. Pharmacists who are specially trained to make custom formulations to meet the requirements of specific doctors and their patients are known as "compounding pharmacists." This practice allows a physician to order a custom-tailored medication not available commercially.

Drug manufacturers must be assured there will be a return on their investment before they commit to developing a new product. To take a new drug from laboratory to licensing can cost hundreds of millions of dollars. The result is that there are limited chemical forms, dosage forms, strengths and flavors available for the physician to prescribe. This can and often does become restrictive for the doctor. Compounding can solve this problem. For example, a patient may be allergic to a preservative or dye in a manufactured product. A compounding pharmacist can prepare the same drug in a preservative-free form.

Most well known these days for providing "bioidentical hormone" preparations, compounding pharmacists are also well versed in the preparation of unique topical formulations for pain. These often consist of using two or more medications with different methods of action in one formula to get a synergistic effect. By combining various medications, smaller concentrations of each medicine can sometimes be used. Compounding also permits pharmacists to prepare small quantities of a prescription which can be used up more quickly to ensure the product maintains its potency for its intended lifespan.

For peripheral neuropathy, a new addition to the treatment of pain is the use of prescription topical gels. A compounding pharmacist will often use a transdermal gel (a form intended for absorption through the skin) as a base or vehicle for the topical application of the active ingredients. The active ingredients can be chosen from a wide range of topical (prilocaine, lidocaine, bupivacaine) or traditionally oral (ketoprofen, indomethacin, amitriptyline, baclofen, clonidine, ketamine, tramadol, gabapentin, Tegretol®) medications.

Although clinical studies of these approaches tend to be small (since there is no drug company licensing the product) there have been a few. In one study, for example, a five-percent ketamine gel applied two to three times daily over the painful skin areas decreased pain significantly in 65 percent of cases of postherpetic neuralgia. Other studies have also found topical gabapentin, amitriptyline and opioids to be effective, on their own and in combination. The beauty of the compounded medication approach is that the medication can be modified to suit the patient. Typically, if results are not seen within one or two weeks the formula can be modified. Compounded analgesics should, however, be used in conjunction with nutritional supplements as opposed to instead of them. Topical analgesics are unlikely to slow nerve damage or increase nerve repair, but they can give welcome symptomatic relief.

Compounded Topical Creams and Gels

The following is a list of common formulations, called transdermal gels that are used to treat neuropathy symptoms:

- Gabapentin and baclofen: As noted in the previous chapter, gabapentin is an anticonvulsant agent that has been shown to have properties that may help block pain receptors. Baclofen is a muscle relaxant and an anti-spasmotic agent.

- Gabapentin and ketamine: Ketamine is an anesthetic agent. The combination of ketamine and gabapentin has been shown to have an analgesic effect.

- Lidocaine, ketamine, and cyclobenzaprine: The analgesic effects of lidocaine and ketamine plus the muscle relaxant action of cyclobenzaprine, has been shown to effectively reduce neuropathic pain in some cases.

- Amitriptyline: This tricyclic antidepressant has been shown to reduce nerve pain when used topically.

These are just some examples of compounded topical gels to treat neuropathic pain. A positive aspect of compounded transdermal gels is that the ingredients along with their respective strengths can be adjusted to meet the needs of patients suffering from peripheral neuropathy.

Special Considerations

Many of the medications that make up transdermal gels are powerful agents when taken orally. Even though only a relatively small amount of these pharmaceutical agents pass through the skin barrier, they can still produce side effects when absorbed in the blood stream. Caution should be used when using any prescription medication, either oral or topical.

There is an organization called the International Academy of Compounding Pharmacists, with more than 1,800 members. Its Web site is http://www.iacprx.org, and its telephone number is 1-800-927-4227. By entering your zip or postal code in the space indicated on the Web site, you can find the names and addresses of local compounding pharmacists in your area.

Non-prescription Creams, Gels, Lotions and Patches

The term for pain, burning and tingling resulting from peripheral neuropathy is called neuropathic pain. Neuropathic pain is not exactly synonymous with sensation of "true pain" but is a way to categorize the extreme discomfort experienced by people with peripheral neuropathy. In many instances the exact opposite holds true in that neuropathy sufferers experience complete numbness with total lack of sensation.

As noted, Lidoderm patches are available by prescription only. Many over-the-counter, non-prescription products have been proven to be effective in reducing the discomfort of peripheral neuropathy. Topical analgesic medications are available as creams, lotions or patches. Some of these medications, such as Neuragen, have been specifically formulated to relieve neuropathic pain. Other products were designed to reduce painful conditions such as arthritis, injuries and back problems and have also proven to successfully treat neuropathy symptoms.

Topical Products Containing Menthol, Methyl Salicylate and Camphor

There are a variety of categories of products used to treat painful areas of the body, with the most common being those containing ingredients of methyl salicylate, menthol and camphor. Methyl salicylate comes from the oil of wintergreen, which is derived from the leaves of the birch tree. Menthol stems from the mint herb. Camphor comes from a combination of plants including peppermint, eucalyptus and cedar.

Methyl salicylate is chemically related to acetylsalicylic acid—better known as aspirin. It is believed that the topical version of aspirin, methyl salicylate, works in a similar fashion to the oral form. In addition to relieving pain, methyl salicylate also seems to produce a warming effect on the skin. This can help "fool" the nerve endings by changing the sensation that one experiences.

Menthol and camphor both have topical anesthetic properties. Studies have shown that the menthol and camphor molecules may have a direct anesthetic effect on the nerve cells responsible for the sensations of pain and temperature perception. Used topically, menthol and camphor appear to dilate the small blood vessels and capillaries that supply the skin. This results in a pleasant warming and pain-relieving sensation.

Precautions When Using these Products

Side effects are uncommon but certain precautions should be taken when using topical creams, gels, lotions and patches. Always use these products in the amounts set forth by the manufacturer. Over-use of these products can lead to toxicity and in very rare instances can be fatal. Some of these topical medications can result in redness, irritation, rashes and blisters when applied to the skin; discontinue use if this should occur. It is important to tell your doctor about any medications, including over-the-counter products, that you are using.

Common Topical Products

There are literally hundreds of products on the market containing a combination of methyl salicylate, menthol and camphor. Some of the more popular products including the ones recommended at the Foot Pain Center are Biofreeze®, Sombra®, Nerve Health + Relief Cream™, Icy Hot®, Flexall®, Mineral Ice® and Aspercreme®.

Ben-Gay patches containing menthol can be applied directly to the area of discomfort and can last up to eight hours. Other patches with varying degrees of combinations of methyl salicylate, menthol and camphor are available as well.

Topical L-Arginine

L-Arginine is an essential amino acid present in the human body. It has a number of important functions including detoxification of ammonia, and assisting the body in the process of protein synthesis, which is important during stressful conditions such as infection, trauma and burns. Topical L-Arginine may play a role in treating peripheral neuropathy pain by its ability to form a compound called nitric oxide. Nitric oxide has a number of important biological functions including blood vessel dilation which helps bring increased blood flow to an area in the body. This compound also plays a role in neurotransmission of certain chemicals for nerve function. As a side note, nitric oxide is responsible for penile erections and is an important part of the process used by the popular drug Viagra®. In most cases the body can produce sufficient amounts of L-Arginine from common dietary sources such vegetable juices, soy and yogurt.

A word of caution: In a study done at Johns Hopkins University, high doses of oral L-Arginine were implicated in increased deaths of those patients recovering from heart attacks.

Side effects from topical L-Arginine are rare since only small amounts are absorbed in to the blood stream. Always follow the directions and dosages as set forth by the manufacturer.

Products Containing Topical L-Arginine

Many companies make topical L-Arginine products with varying percentages of this compound. It may be found in pharmacies, local health stores or on the Internet. A product used and recommended at the Foot Pain Center is called Healthibetic™.

Topical botanical products

Topical botanical products are derived from the ingredients contained in plants. Many topical botanicals are used in cosmetic products to moisturize and repair skin damage caused by the sun and pollutants. Some botanical agents have been shown to be effective in reducing pain and inflammation. The analgesic properties of some topical agents make them useful in the treatment of neuropathic pain. Most botanicals have a long history of safety. Certain topicals—especially when ingested, such as sassafras have been banned as food additives due to potential toxicity. Side effects and adverse reaction to topical botanical products are rare.

Advantages of Topical Medications

- Topical medications are quick acting. Analgesic creams and gels can literally work in seconds to help relieve neuropathic pain. As noted, these medications can be extremely helpful at night when symptoms often are the worst. Similarly if you experience an "attack" or a sudden flare-up of symptoms during the day, by applying a cream or gel you may be able to break the pain cycle and avoid further discomfort.

- Topical medications have fewer side effects than oral drugs used for treating peripheral neuropathy. It is estimated that only a very small percentage of ingredients in topical medications actually cross the skin barrier and are absorbed into the bloodstream. All topicals should be used as directed. Even seemingly innocuous creams and gels that contain ingredients like menthol can cause serious side effects if used in excess.

- Topicals can "spot treat" certain areas in the body that are particularly uncomfortable. It may not be necessary to use an oral medication if you experience neuropathic pain in a localized area. Some people with peripheral neuropathy may experience burning or tingling in just one or two toes. In such cases a topical product may be sufficient to control the discomfort.

- Topical medications are non-habit forming.

Disadvantages of Topical Medications

- Only a small amount of medication penetrates through the skin barrier, limiting its effectiveness. This is an advantage in reducing side effects; however it is a disadvantage in that only a minimal dosage of the medication is actually absorbed into the system.

- Topical medications may not penetrate deep to nerve tissue. Even superficial nerves lie many centimeters below the skin surface. The deep nerves in the feet and leg, such as the peroneal nerve, are situated even deeper below the skin. Since the skin on the feet and legs—in particular on the palms and soles—is so thick, penetration to levels of these nerves is not always possible.

- Choosing an effective topical medication is usually a "trial and error" process. Many of the analgesic creams, gels and patches are not targeted to specifically treat peripheral neuropathy pain. Many have been formulated to treat generalized pains such as arthritic pain, injuries and shingles (postherpetic neuralgia). As analgesic agents they may be helpful in reducing neuropathic pain, but a degree of experimentation is often necessary to determine which ones, if any, are effective in reducing pain, tingling or burning symptoms often associated with peripheral neuropathy.

- Analgesic effects of topical products are usually short-acting. Once absorbed through the skin, topicals may only work for very limited periods of time. Transdermal patches (which will be discussed in this chapter) are time-released and are longer acting.

Chapter 7

Nutrients for Neuropathy

"In my opinion, the best thing most PNers could do is begin a sensible program of nutrient supplementation." – John A. Senneff, author of "Numb Toes and Aching Soles"

Introduction

It has long been known that deficiencies of nutrients can be the cause of disease. Scurvy (vitamin C deficiency) and pellagra (vitamin B3 deficiency) are often cited examples of this phenomenon. Although often intuitively understood by the average person, scientists only now are discovering that suboptimal levels of nutrients may contribute to less-than-optimal health and vitality and leave the body vulnerable to the onset of chronic disease. We live in an era when less than 20 percent of North Americans consume the recommended amounts of fruits and vegetables. At the same time, environmental pollution, stress, drugs and chemicals added to foods all deplete important nutrients from our bodies. Even the foods we consume, which are grown in nutrient-depleted soils using chemical fertilizers and pesticides, are suspect in terms of their ability to provide adequate nutrition. Although it has not been proven scientifically, it seems likely that the increased rates of chronic disease are in part due to nutrient deficiencies. This applies to neuropathies in particular, since nervous tissue is one type of tissue in the body that is very sensitive to toxins and nutrient deficiencies (such as B12 deficiency, which is known to cause neuropathy) and has limited capacity for repair.

The purpose of this chapter is to explore some of the most important nutrients for the prevention of neuropathy, and for the best chances of optimizing nerve repair and preventing neuropathies from worsening. Keep in mind that, due to the nature of nerve cells and the fact that nutrients are not pain killers, one should use nutritional supplementation for about three months before deciding if there is any benefit. If someone were to show even a 10 to 20 percent improvement in symptoms over three months that is very encouraging, since chances are they would likely have shown a worsening of symptoms with no treatment. It is also encouraging because often improvements continue past three months if the neuropathy sufferer is diligent about maintaining the supplement regime.

Lipoic Acid

Lipoic acid is a very much investigated nutrient for diabetic neuropathy and provided the first clear evidence that nutritional treatment can reverse the course of neuropathy. At least 15 controlled and randomized clinical trials of lipoic acid in patients with diabetic neuropathy have been performed using different study designs, durations of treatment, doses, sample sizes, and patient populations. Also known as "alpha-lipoic acid," it is a powerful free radical scavenger found in the cells of humans and in a variety of foods. It has been called a universal antioxidant because it is both fat- and water-soluble, and it has also been shown to recycle other antioxidants, such as vitamins E and C. Lipoic acid has also been used to reverse damage associated with mushroom poisoning, radiation, alcoholic hepatitis, and heavy metal toxicity.

Lipoic acid is approved in Germany for clinical use in the management of diabetic polyneuropathy, and it has been used for this purpose in Europe for decades. A systematic review done in Germany of 15 trials concluded that short-term treatment with alpha-lipoic acid, 600 mg/day, reduces the symptoms of diabetic neuropathy. Statistically significant improvements in pain, tingling, and numbness compared with placebo were seen at this dose in a number of trials. Depletion of lipoic acid has also been documented in persons with diabetes with neuropathies. Research on lipoic acid supplementation has also shown improvements in glucose metabolism, reduced glycosylation of proteins (such as HbA1c), improved blood flow to peripheral nerves, and stimulation of nerve cell conduction. In one study, treatment with lipoic acid improved the efficiency with which insulin worked by 27 percent in only four weeks.

Clinical studies to date have indicated that alpha-lipoic acid is generally safe and well-tolerated with minimal side effects. Although lipoic acid has not been proven to be beneficial for non-diabetic forms of neuropathy, its mechanism of action suggests it is worth trying for neuropathies from all causes. Adverse effects tend to be mild and include headache, skin rash, and stomach upset at high doses (>600 mg/day). In some cases these effects may be due to the detoxification process; consuming plenty of water and vitamin C at 2,000 to 6,000 mg per day may help the symptoms to resolve.

Methylcobalamin

Methylcobalamin is the active form of vitamin B12. Cyanocobalamin, another form of B12, is the most widely available and least expensive form of this B vitamin, and is found in most over-the-counter multivitamins. However, cyanocobalamin is an inactive precursor that must be converted into one of two active metabolites: methylcobalamin and adenosylcobalamin. Of these two, methylcobalamin seems to be the most neurologically active. Studies have suggested that methylcobalamin is better utilized by the body and better retained in tissue than cyanocobalamin. The clinical experience of many health care practitioners seems to further support the use of the methylcobalamin form for nerve-related conditions.

Vitamin B12 plays a critical role in the maintenance of nerve myelin, and it is well known that prolonged B12 deficiency in healthy individuals can lead to nerve degeneration and irreversible neurological damage.

In experimental models, high doses of B12 in the methylcobalmin form has been shown to increase nerve regeneration. It has also been shown to decrease the neuropathic pain experienced by a group of patients with kidney failure. It has also been found that HIV patients with neuropathy statistically have lower B12 levels than those HIV patients who do not suffer from this condition. In a small study, adding B12 injections to the treatment program of HIV patients resulted in improvements in symptoms in five of eight patients within one week of treatment.

The recommended dosage for clinical effects is 5 to 15 mg per day (yes, milligrams) of methylcobalamin, taken orally (sublingually), intramuscularly, or intravenously. Positive clinical results have been reported irrespective of the method of administration. Methylcobalamin has excellent tolerability and no known toxicity. Alcohol, antibiotics, oral diabetes medications, beta blockers, anti-acid drugs (H2 blockers), oral contraceptives, nicotine, and HIV drugs can also cause vitamin B12 depletion.

Vitamin E

Oxidative stress (free radical damage) appears to play a significant role in the development of peripheral neuropathy. Vitamin E is an antioxidant which protects cells from free radical damage. Diets high in vitamin E have been shown to be protective against many health conditions, and vitamin E deficiency is a known and proven cause of peripheral neuropathy. For instance, vitamin E deficiency is known to cause neuropathy in patients who have undergone gastrectomy (removal of part or all of the stomach) and likely any other causes of mal-absorption of fat soluble vitamins such as inflammatory bowel conditions.

When supplementing vitamin E, it is important to get the right form. The best forms are known as "natural, mixed tocopherol" forms of vitamin E which contains a variety of naturally occurring vitamin E molecules designated as "d," as in "d-alpha-tocopherol." Avoid synthetic forms which are labeled "dl" as in "dl-alpha-tocopherol."

Vitamin E has been studied in diabetic peripheral neuropathy (see diabetes chapter), the prevention of chemotherapy-induced neuropathy, and post-gastrectomy neuropathy. Vitamin E was shown to prevent the development of PN from at least two chemotherapy drugs, cisplatin and paclitaxel, without negatively affecting their efficacy. In another study of 10 patients with post-gastrectomy neuropathies, nine patients reported improvement with 150 to 300 mg of vitamin E daily.

Multi-B Vitamins

Considering that the B vitamin group affects many aspects of cell metabolism and therefore healthy nerve functioning, it may be more effective to supplement the entire group of B vitamins. A combination of B1, B6 and B12 was tested in an animal model of neuropathic pain. In this case, recovery from pain was rated as 20 percent to 100 percent at 12 hours, with recovery being twice as fast as a saline (salt) placebo. Overall, the B vitamin combination reduced both the severity and duration of pain. In these animal studies, results were likely more pronounced than in the human multi-B vitamin trials because neuropathy was induced immediately prior to treatment, as opposed to typical neuropathy in humans which takes years to develop and usually is present a long time before treatment is initiated. Nevertheless, including a multiple-B vitamin seems a prudent approach to maximizing the potential for nerve repair, especially for anyone taking pharmaceutical drugs for pain, which are known to deplete B vitamin levels.

Folate

If taking a multi-B vitamin, or a combination product, make sure it contains the important nutrient folic acid or folate. A deficiency of folate has been associated with the development of PN in a number of surveys. Neuropathies also can be caused by a variety of medications known to create folate deficiency, including sulfa antibiotics, methotrexate, anti-tuberculosis drugs, anticonvulsants and birth control pills. Folate, of course, is the nutrient recommended for all pregnant women because it prevents spinal cord defects by contributing to healthy cell division. Without healthy levels of this important nutrient, it is very difficult for nerve cells to regenerate and repair. At least 400 mcg of folate should be consumed daily.

Biotin

Biotin is another nutrient often found in multi-B vitamins and combination products. Biotin supplementation has been shown to be beneficial for uremic (kidney failure-induced) neuropathy and for diabetic neuropathy. A reasonable daily intake of biotin is 5 mg per day.

Inositol

Inositol is an important constituent of nerve cell membranes. Low levels of inositol have been implicated in the development of PN, including diabetic neuropathy. Diets high in inositol—foods such as cantaloupe, peanuts, grapefruit, and whole grains—have been shown to improve diabetic neuropathy. Researchers at the University of Alabama found a statistically significant improvement in nerve function in persons with diabetes placed on a diet high in inositol. In other research, supplementation with inositol in doses of 2 to 6 grams per day has resulted in improvements in neuropathy.

Essential Fatty Acids

Essential fatty acids (EFAs) are fat-soluble acids that must be obtained from the diet because they are, in fact, essential for healthy human metabolism, including healthy nerve function. There are two essential fatty acids in human nutrition: omega-3 and omega-6. They are often consumed in the diet as linolenic and linoleic acid. However, these fatty acids require an enzyme called delta-6-desaturase to convert into their useful forms. Delta-6-desaturase converts linolenic acid to eicosapentaenoic acid (EPA) and linoleic acid to Gamma-Linolenic acid (GLA). This conversion process is often severely compromised in many people for a variety of reasons including low thyroid function, diabetes or over-reliance on refined carbohydrates, and toxic exposures. Since EPA, DHA (Docosahexaenoic Acid, an omega-3 fat found in fish oils) and GLA are essential for healthy nerve cell function, it makes sense to supplement these two oils directly. It is therefore recommended that those with PN supplement with an EPA/DHA blend at a daily dose of 1,800 mg of EPA and 900 mg DHA as well as at least 300 mg per day of GLA.

Magnesium

The common mineral magnesium is an essential cofactor in human metabolism, assisting more than 300 chemical reactions including the conversion of glucose to energy. Magnesium deficiency has been associated with high blood pressure, diabetes, high cholesterol, cardiovascular disease, and complications of pregnancy. Since magnesium is a common nutrient deficiency in North America, and since magnesium is needed by every cell in the body including neurons to produce energy, supplementation with magnesium is recommended. Other factors which deplete magnesium include diabetes, medications (especially diuretics for high blood pressure) malabsorption syndromes of the gastrointestinal tract, low stomach acid (hypochlorhydria), diets low in minerals, and alcohol and caffeine use.

Doses of 300 to 600 mg per day of magnesium citrate are appropriate for patients with normal kidney function. Magnesium therapy should be undertaken only with the guidance of a health care practitioner familiar with its use. Good dietary sources include whole grains, leafy green vegetables, legumes, nuts, and fish. Organic sources of these foods have been shown to be as much as 10 times higher in minerals versus conventionally farmed versions. Note also that diets high in saturated fat, sugar, fructose, caffeine, and alcohol may increase magnesium requirements.

Carnitine

Carnitine, also known as L-carnitine or acetyl-l-carnitine, is an amino acid-like compound which is synthesized from two amino acids, lysine and methionine, primarily in the liver and kidneys. Carnitine helps in the metabolism of fat in the body because it is responsible for transporting fatty acids into the fat-burning compartment of the cells. It has been shown that during growth, pregnancy, or disease there may be a deficiency of carnitine available. Carnitine levels have been shown to be lower in people with diabetic PN.

Carnitine, given as a nutritional supplement, has been shown to be beneficial for a number of neuropathies including diabetic neuropathy (see diabetes chapter), HIV neuropathy and chemo-therapy-induced neuropathy. In 21 patients with HIV-induced neuropathy, carnitine given at a dose of 1,500 mg twice daily resulted in improvement in 76 percent of patients. The treatment was continued for up to 33 months but biopsies of the skin showed increased nerve function within six months. Carnitine also has been shown in a number of small trials to improve neuropathy caused by the chemotherapy drugs taxanes (pacli-taxel, docetaxel) and platinums (cisplatin, oxaliplatin, carbopla-tin) and vinca alkaloids (vinblastine, vincristine). In animal studies, carnitine has also been shown to help prevent neuropathy if taken along with the chemotherapeutic agent and does not seem to interfere with the anti-tumor effects of the drugs.

The recommended dose of carnitine is 1g per day.

Nutrient Name	Recommended Daily Dose	Function	Studied in
Lipoic Acid	600–1200 mg	Antioxidant, water and fat soluble	Diabetic neuropathy
Methylcobalamin	5–15 mg sublingually or injection	Nerve regeneration	HIV neuropathy
Vitamin E	400 mg per day of mixed tocopherol form	Antioxidant	Diabetic neuropathy Post-gastrectomy neuropathy Chemotherapy-induced neuropathy
Multi-B Vitamin	50–100 mg	Healthy nerve function	Pain relief of induced neuropathy in animal studies
Folate	400 ug to 1 mg	Healthy cell division	Deficiency associated with neuropathy
Biotin	5 mg	Nerve cell health	Kidney failure-induced neuropathy
Inositol	2–6 g	Nerve cell membrane	Diabetic neuropathy
Essential Fatty Acids	• EPA 1800 mg • DHA 900 mg • GLA 300 mg	Component of nerve myelin	Diabetic neuropathy
Magnesium	300–600 mg	Nerve cell energy production	Deficiency is common especially in persons with diabetes
Carnitine	1 g		Diabetic neuropathy, HIV neuropathy and chemotherapy-induced neuropathy

Table 3: Summary of Nutrients for Neuropathy & Recommended Daily Dose

The Numb Foot Book

Chapter 8

East Meets West: Tai Chi and Acupuncture

Tai Chi

"Next to making certain we are receiving the proper nutrients in an adequate amount, the most important thing a PNer can do is exercise." – John A. Senneff

One form of exercise mentioned by John A. Senneff in the original "Numb Toes" is the Chinese martial arts routine called tai chi. This is a training exercise involving slow, graceful movements that are derived from the movements of animals and follow a natural, relaxed pattern. They increase the body's range of motion and are said to exercise the internal organs. According to practitioners, the slow meditative routine aids stress reduction and promotes relaxation, improved balance and better posture, while increasing blood flow.

Since the publication of the original Numb Toes, Dr. Li Li of Louisiana State University (LSU) has been studying the effect of physical activity on people with peripheral neuropathy. The LSU Peripheral Neuropathy Studies have investigated a number of exercises, including tai chi, assisted walking, and focused exercise. Dr. Li has published a number of interesting results from these

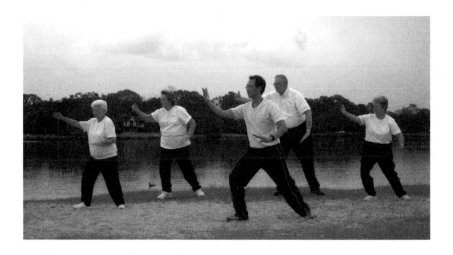

programs including reduced pain, improved sensation, improved balance, better ability to walk, and maybe most important of all, better quality of life.

Dr. Li, a kinesiologist (specialist in the study of movement and gait), became interested in the unique problems posed by peripheral neuropathy when he noticed an LSU facility services worker using a cane in a unique way. "Charlie" carried a cane but he did not use it to walk, only to stand. When Dr. Li asked why, Charlie told him that he had a condition called peripheral neuropathy. Dr. Li was confused because conventional medical teaching implies that one cannot walk if one cannot stand.

Dr. Li began his neuropathy study in 2004. Now, he has approximately 75 individuals enrolled, with groups meeting three times a week for tai chi lessons. The tai chi exercises have been modified to suit people with peripheral neuropathy. They are even slower than what you would find in the general public market for tai chi exercise classes. Participants started with a modified beginner's class, many of them holding onto chairs to keep their balance. Classes were typically two to three times a week for 60-minute sessions. Remarkably, weeks later in the sessions there were "no more chairs," says Dr. Li. In fact, Dr. Li's classes have become so popular that there are over 150 people on a waiting list for admittance.

As noted in the comments from participants, the results that Dr. Li and his team are seeing are encouraging. Many people start the program unable to stand up for more than five minutes at a time. Yet, after as few as six weeks, many of them can stand unassisted for long periods of time. Many of these people were previously told to expect to be in wheelchairs by this point. Dr. Li believes that the tai chi training improves dynamic balance. He also believes that continued practice increases awareness of the body's position and orientation, helping PNer's take control of their balance and prevent falls. As a result, many participants are back to doing things they used to take for granted, like being able to stand in a shower and wash their hair with their eyes closed.

These results are confirmed by Dr. Li using standardized testing such as balance, timed get-up-and-go, mobility and knee strength tests. For example, the mobility test involves nonstop walking for six minutes and the timed get-up-and-go test measures the overall time taken to complete a series of functionally important tasks. Overall, Dr. Li has found that practicing tai chi exercises can result in far greater levels of improvement than pursuing more conventional methods of treatment. To rule out the placebo effect, Dr. Li compared tai chi to other types of interventions including strength training, walking and infrared light therapy. So far tai chi is still the undisputed winner.

Exactly how tai chi benefits neuropathy sufferers is not clear. Dr. Li believes there might be a link between tai chi and nerve re-growth. Many of his participants have been able to give up their canes and walkers. One participant reported that after two weeks he could feel his toes again, something he had not been able to do for the previous five years. Dr. Li's preliminary results indicate there might be a link between tai chi and nerve growth, and he hopes more studies will prove a definite connection.

"(Tai chi) makes me feel better and helps me with my balance."

   - AC, 20 yr sufferer of PN

"To those people out there with peripheral neuropathy, I definitely recommend this type of program to them."

   - ES, active and healthy PN sufferer

"(Tai chi) makes my numbness go away and it feels better, even my toes and my balance has improved."

   - MO, 71-year-old woman with PN

"I feel much better when I am walking or doing (tai chi) exercises. I don't feel the pain in my feet as much when I am moving or active."

   - JF, woman with seven year history of PN

Acupuncture

Acupuncture has been documented as being in use in China as early as 2697 B.C. According to classical Chinese theory, the important factor in maintaining pain-free health is assuring that our body energy, called qi, is unimpeded and flows smoothly. According to this view, channels of qi, called meridians, run in ordered patterns throughout the body. Obstructions in the meridians cause deficiencies of energy, blood and nerve pulses, eventually leading to disease. Traditional Chinese medicine teaches that one cause of peripheral neuropathy is "dampness moving to the limbs, where it obstructs the flow of qi (energy) and blood." Very thin stainless steel needles properly placed at designated points, and sometimes twirled or to which an electric current or heat is sometimes supplied, are thought to unblock the channels. According to this theory, acupuncture treatments restore the regular flow of qi to a particular body, promoting health and relieving pain.

An acupuncturist who practices in the traditional manner will do an interview and ask questions about how, where and when you feel pain, as well as inquire about other seemingly unrelated symptoms such as perspiration, sleep, bowel and urination habits. The practitioner may also feel the pulse and observe the tongue for clues as to where the qi is obstructed. Each patient is then custom-treated with a unique set of acupuncture points, many of which are on the hands and feet, according to his or her specific symptoms and Chinese medicine diagnosis. In addition to acupuncture, other methods of treatment such as herbal and physical therapy may be suggested to achieve faster results.

People are often afraid to try acupuncture because of the belief that all needles are by nature painful. However, most people feel little sensitivity to the insertion of the acupuncture needles. This is because the acupuncture needles are so thin. Occasionally, there is a brief moment of discomfort as the needle penetrates the skin. This may be followed by a slight heaviness, achiness or even analgesic effect. Once all the needles are in place, the patient is typically instructed to relax for 20 to 30 minutes. Many people even fall asleep during that time. The length, number and frequency of treatments will vary with the individual, but in general more severe or chronic ailments often require more treatments. In China, the frequency of treatment is much greater, with people being treated every day in some cases. In North America it is more common to see people receiving weekly or twice-a-week treatments.

The Western "scientific" explanation is that acupuncture needles stimulate nerves and cause certain chemicals to be released in the muscles, spinal cord and brain. For example, one class of chemical compounds called endorphins has been shown to be released from acupuncture treatments. Endorphins are very potent naturally occurring pain killers in the body, which work in the same way as morphine. Over the course of a number of treatments the release of other chemicals and hormones influences the body's own pain regulating system, hopefully leading to a down regulation of pain signals.

Acupuncture has grown tremendously in popularity in the West. In the April 1, 1998, issue of the prestigious journal, Nature, the following comment was made:

"Research has shown that acupuncture has relieved pain in 70 percent of [people] who have sought treatment. Clinical trials show acupuncture is successful in treating osteoarthritis of the knee, tennis elbow, headaches, facial and back pain. In the United States alone, one million people use acupuncture each year."

The World Health Organization has gone on record as stating that several groups of diseases, including peripheral neuropathy, respond well to acupuncture treatment.

Clinical Research

There have been a number of clinical trials examining acupuncture's efficacy in providing PN pain relief. A study performed at the University of Manchester, U. K., in 1998 looked at acupuncture for the treatment of chronic peripheral diabetic neuropathy. Forty-six patients received up to six courses of classical acupuncture over a period of 10 weeks, using traditional Chinese acupuncture points. Forty-four completed the study with 34 (77 percent) showing significant improvement in their symptoms. These results were followed up for a period of 18 to 52 weeks with 67 percent saying they were able to stop or reduce their medications significantly. Seven, in fact, noted their symptoms cleared completely. The researchers concluded that "acupuncture is a safe and effective therapy for the long-term management of painful diabetic neuropathy, although its mechanism of action remains speculative."

More recent clinical trials have shown that acupuncture can improve nerve conduction. For example, as reported in the European Journal of Neurology, among 47 patients who met the criteria for PN (of unknown cause), 21 patients received acupuncture therapy according to classical Chinese Medicine, while 26 patients received the best medical care but no specific treatment for PN. Sixteen patients (76 percent) in the acupuncture group had improvements in symptoms and objective improvements in nerve conduction speed. Only four patients in the no-acupuncture group had improvements. The data suggested to the researchers that "there is a positive effect of acupuncture on PN of undefined etiology (cause) as measured by objective parameters."

European Journal of Neurology
Volume 14 Issue 3 Page 276-281, March 2007
To cite this article: S. Schröder, J. Liepert, A. Remppis, J. H. Greten (2007) Acupuncture treatment improves nerve conduction in peripheral neuropathy European Journal of Neurology 14 (3), 276–281.
doi:10.1111/j.1468-1331.2006.01632.x

Mother of two develops neuropathic pain after car accident

Monica, a 36-year-old mother of two young boys, was beside herself with frustration and had difficulty even describing her circumstance. Three years previously, as the result of a serious car accident, she was experiencing chronic "electric" pain in her low back. The pain was so intense ("10 out of 10") that she rarely slept for more than one hour at a time and more than four hours each night. Yet, her insurance company had deemed that she was ready to return to full-time administrative work, based on the fact that X-rays and MRI scans had revealed no evidence of permanent damage, as is often the case with neuropathic pain. Yet, no medications except strong narcotics, prescribed by the local pain clinic, had even blunted her pain. In addition, Monica was suffering from extreme nausea, vomiting and diarrhea with lack of appetite brought on, she believed, by her medications, especially gabapentin. She had lost 24 pounds in six months and was down to 116 pounds. Mostly, she was concerned that her children were suffering from the loss of their mother.

Treatment

A treatment protocol was devised for Monica consisting of digestive support (probiotics, enzymes and powdered nutrient mix), a topical natural analgesic for pain (Neuragen®), a vitamin B-12 injection, an herbal stress tonic (Adaptogen from WTSmed.com), and melatonin tablets to aid in sleep. As well, a weekly acupuncture treatment program was begun. After one acupuncture treatment Monica reported three days of pain reduction down to seven (on a one to 10 scale). On the next visit Monica reported the first regular bowel movement that she had experienced in one year. The topical analgesic applied three times a day, had helped her manage her pain, and her sleep was up to three hours uninterrupted. Her overall energy had improved to four (on a scale of one to 100) up from previously rating her energy a two (on a scale of one to 10).

One month after beginning treatments Monica reported that she was able to achieve six to seven hours per night of restful sleep for the first time in years, and her energy was now six (on a scale of one to 10) during the day. She was able to discontinue all her pharmaceutical medications and her average pain declined to a rating of five (on a scale of one to 10). Eventually, Monica was able to return to part-time work and now manages her condition with these approaches, the occasional acupuncture treatment, as well as by avoiding overworking or getting overtired.

Chapter 9

Walking and Balance Problems

As explained in previous chapters, peripheral neuropathy causes disturbances in sensation, including, pain, numbness, burning and tingling. When damage to the motor nerves (the nerves that control muscle stimulation and muscle movement) occurs, walking and balance problems frequently arise. Walking or gait problems range from minor disturbances such as a slight unsteadiness to severe and debilitating walking difficulties. The causes of gait and balance problems along with solutions will be discussed in this chapter. To have a better understanding of the impact of peripheral neuropathy on gait and balance, actual cases from the Foot Pain Center will be presented first.

Case 1 "ST" 66-year-old female

"I use to love to walk and now I dread it because I am so unsteady on my feet.

I used to walk everywhere. I would walk with my lady friends around the neighborhood three or four times a week. On weekends, I would go shopping with my husband and stand and walk for hours at a time. Now I avoid walking as much as possible. I am very unsteady and I feel like I have to hold onto something to keep myself from falling."

Case 2 "AW" 71-year-old female

"I lose my balance when I walk and have fallen a few times. Once I fell and broke my arm.

I lose my balance when I am walking and have tripped and fallen on about four occasions. Once when I was going to the bathroom in the middle of the night, I completely lost my balance and fell on my right arm. In the morning I noticed that my arm was very swollen. I went to the emergency room and the x-ray showed that I had broken my arm. I was placed in a cast for six weeks. Now I am scared to walk for fear that I might fall again. People have told me that I am lucky that I have not broken a hip."

Case 3 "LD" 70-year-old male

"I am very self-conscious about the way I walk. I drift to the side and can't seem to walk in a straight line.

About 10 years ago, I was diagnosed with peripheral neuropathy. I get tingling and the feeling of electric shocks shooting into my toes. A few years after I was told I had peripheral neuropathy I noticed I had problems walking. I seem to teeter and walk crooked. I cannot walk in a straight path. I am 70-years-old and my grown children tell me to try to walk straighter. If I concentrate really hard I can do it for a few steps but I soon go back to walking the way I usually do. It is very frustrating."

Case 4 "SW" 61-year-old male

My feet and legs get tired so easy that it feels like I have lead weights attached to them.

I can't even walk one block before my feet and legs get so tired that I have to sit down. I also hate going up and down stairs. I live in a two-story house. I can hardly make it up the first landing. I usually have to stop and rest before moving on."

Case 5 "DS" 77-year-old female

"I get terrible cramping and soreness in my feet and legs."

I am very unsteady when I walk. It takes a great effort just to keep myself upright and by the end of the day and in the evening I get aching and cramping in my feet and legs.

I am so unsteady when I walk it seems to take all my strength just to keep myself upright. I can feel myself putting strain on my feet, legs, knees and my hips. It even hurts in my lower back when I walk. After a few hours my muscles get very sore. Even when I am off my feet in the evenings I experience aching and cramping in my feet and legs."

Case 6 "LG" 58-year-old female

"I drag my feet when I walk. I can't pick them up and I find walking almost impossible.

It started about eight years ago. At first I noticed that I shuffled my feet and had difficulty raising them up and down when I walked. My husband would always remind me to pick up my feet when I walked. I was able to pick them up if I really concentrated. Over the next few years, I completely lost the ability to pick my feet up when I walk. Even when I am off my feet they dangle in a downwards position. I have been diagnosed with drop foot. I wear braces on my legs which is a great help when I walk."

Why People with Peripheral Neuropathy Have Walking and Balance Problems

There are many reasons why peripheral neuropathy sufferers have walking difficulties. In previous chapters it was noted that neuropathy is a condition that affects both the sensory and motor nerves. Sensory nerves supply feeling to the feet; motor nerves allow movement of the muscles of the feet and legs. When one loses the ability to feel his/her feet, balance can be severely affected. The brain and spinal cord, which are the computers of the central nervous system, are not properly communicating with the lower extremities. The brain sends signals to the feet, which allow the feet to adjust to a variety of factors. As we move from one surface to another—for example from a hard cement sidewalk to a soft and uneven grassy lawn—the brain will allow us to compensate for these changes. If people have lost feeling in their feet, they lose this ability and are more prone to unsteadiness and falling.

No one likes to experience pain! Yet pain is an important protective mechanism for our bodies. For example, if we sprain our ankle, the brain sends pain signals and our natural reaction is to avoid putting pressure on this area. This can prevent further injury to the area. People with nerve damage often lose this ability, which is referred to as *loss of protective sensation.*

This can cause severe balance problems and also may cause serious injury to the skin, bones, joints, tendons and ligaments of the feet. If a person without nerve damage puts excessive pressure on a particular bone or joint in the foot, the pain factor "kicks in" and this person will consciously or unconsciously shift his/her weight to avoid further injury. Since many people with peripheral neuropathy cannot feel their feet, they may continue walking on this problem area thus causing additional injury.

In extreme cases, a loss of protective sensation can cause a serious medical condition called Charcot foot. Charcot foot is a complication of peripheral neuropathy, frequently seen in persons with diabetes. This condition results in weakness of the bones and joints which often leads to multiple fractures in the metatarsals and other bones in the foot. As the bones continue to weaken, the arch can collapse, making it even more difficult to walk.

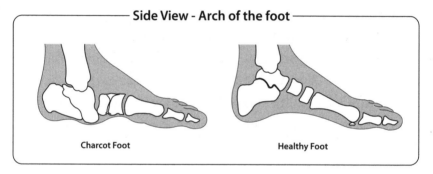

Fig. 10: Charcot Foot

Symptoms of Charcot-Marie-Tooth disease include:

- Swelling of the foot, especially in the inside and bottom of the foot

- Redness and inflammation in the foot

- Throbbing and burning

- Foot feels warm to touch

- "Shooting pains" and aching in the foot

Treating Charcot foot can be quite involved. Rest and im-mobilization are extremely important. This helps prevent further bone and joint damage. Immobilization is accomplished by keeping the patient off his/her feet as much as possible. The patient is usually placed in a below the knee cast or, in some cases, surgery is required to realign the damaged foot. When the inflammation and bone destruction are sufficiently controlled, the next phase of treatment includes the dispensing of modified and custom shoes. This will be discussed later in this chapter.

Odd Sensations Contribute to Balance Problems

Peripheral neuropathy patients at the Foot Pain Center describe these sensations in many ways—the feeling of walking on sand-paper, cardboard, rocks, marbles or pins are just a few. When people have the sensation of walking on rocks or marbles, it does interfere with the normal walking pattern. A person who experiences these sensations is distracted when walking and cannot effectively concentrate on the normal heel-to-toe gait.

Loss of Proprioception: Ability to Know Where Your Feet are Positioned Relative to the Ground

Proprioception is often referred to as the sixth sense. Our brain sends out impulses and allows us to sense where a particular body part is situated without visually seeing it. A test that has been previously described is called the propioceptive sensation test. This test consists of having a patient sit in an examination chair with eyes closed. The examiner moves a body part, usually the great toe in upward or downward position. A person with adequate proprioceptive ability can differentiate the different positions of the toe.

It is extremely important for good balance to be able to sense where your feet are situated at all times. Picture an astronaut floating around in his space vehicle. Without the sensation of "being grounded" it is most difficult to remain orientated to your surroundings. The same holds true for a person with peripheral neuropathy. If this person does not feel where his/her feet are relative to the ground, unsteadiness and imbalance will occur.

Muscle Weakness as a Cause of Balance Problems

Motor nerves carry impulses from skeletal muscles which creates voluntary movement. For example, when we want to move our pinky finger, the brain sends impulses to the muscle fibers around the pinky. This results in muscle contraction which then causes the finger to move. People with peripheral neuropathy often have damage to these motor nerves. The impulses that stimulate muscles may be weak or absent. This can result in loss of muscle function. In order to walk properly and with good balance, the muscles of the feet and legs must have sufficient strength to support our body weight, propel us forward and counteract the forces of gravity. The degree of nerve damage is proportional to the amount of difficulty one experiences during walking. Mild damage to the motor nerves may result in weakness and fatigue. People with motor nerve damage may only be able to walk for short distances before experiencing pain and fatigue. They may have difficulty walking up a flight of steps or going up and down hills.

Moderate motor nerve damage will invariably cause greater walking difficulties. Weakness of the muscles of the feet and legs will often cause a person to shuffle his or her feet. Another problem that can occur is drifting to one side when walking. Many muscles have an opposing muscle or muscle group having equal strength that pulls in the opposite direction. For example, muscles that are responsible for extension of the knee have an opposing muscle group causing flexion of the knee. A person possessing healthy, functioning nerves will have an equal push-pull of these opposing muscles. When one muscle is weak and is not adequately stimulated by the motor nerves, the opposing muscle will over-power the other one. This results in imbalance and instability.

Severe motor nerve damage will result in major walking difficulties. In cases where nerve damage is so advanced, the muscle may not receive any nerve impulses. In these instances the muscle will not contract at all. Severe nerve damage in the lower extremities can result in partial or complete paralysis. A condition called drop foot deformity is often due to severe motor nerve damage.

Drop Foot Deformity

Drop foot (also known as foot drop) is a condition caused by severe weakness of the muscles around the ankle joint. With drop foot, a person loses the ability to raise the foot at the ankle. This causes severe instability when walking. Drop foot is treated by using braces and other devices and will be discussed in detail later in this chapter.

Not All Balance Problems Are Due To Peripheral Neuropathy

As noted, peripheral neuropathy can definitely cause walking problems yet there are many other conditions that may also have a detrimental effect on gait and balance. The inner ear is responsible for maintaining balance. Vestibular (inner ear) problems can cause imbalance and vertigo. Vertigo is a feeling that you or your surroundings are moving when in fact, there is no actual movement. People with vertigo may experience feelings of falling, spinning or tilting to one side. Multiple sclerosis is a central nervous system disorder. Multiple sclerosis is a chronic disease that can cause a variety of symptoms including muscle weakness and problems with balance.

Parkinson's disease is a degenerative disease of the central nervous system that often causes severe walking difficulties. People with Parkinson's disease usually have a "shuffling gait" which is characterized by short steps. The feet barely leave the ground, making walking a challenge. These people are more prone to tripping on the smallest of objects.

Other causes of walking and balance problems include:

- Degenerative muscle disease such as muscular dystrophy

- Arthritis

- Stroke

- Spinal cord injury, spinal stenosis and herniated-slipped disc

Treating Walking and Balance Problems

An important goal in treating gait and balance problems is to keep the person active. People with peripheral neuropathy who are unsteady on their feet or have a history of falling, tend to shy away from walking but leading an active life-style is extremely beneficial in countering the effects of nerve damage. Walking helps prevent muscle atrophy (muscle wasting) and can actually build up muscle tone. Being able to walk even on a limited basis, can help increase localized circulation. Of course walking can greatly benefit the cardiovascular system, can help reduce cholesterol levels, and lower blood pressure in those people who are hypertensive.

On the contrary, a more sedentary life style can exacerbate many medical problems. Inactivity leads to muscle weakness and atrophy. This will start a negative cycle leading to greater muscle weakness, which makes walking even more difficult, thus leading to further problems. People who are bedridden tend to be prone to infections of the feet and pressure (decubitus) ulcers.

Advancements in the field of kinesiology—the study of human motion, have made walking and balance problems more treatable. There is no one magic bullet to improve gait and balance as it usually takes a combination of treatments. Goals for the patient with balance difficulties must be realistic. A person who is very unsteady and can only walk for very short distances should strive for gradual improvement.

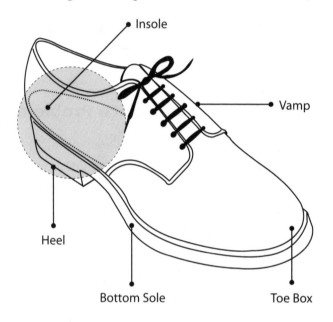

Fig. 11: Components of a Shoe

Ways to Improve Walking and Balance

Walking Aids: Canes and walkers

Many people are resistant to using canes or walkers, having the belief that there is a stigma attached to using such devices. Using a walking aid is a good first step in gaining confidence when walking. Walking outside the home, particularly in crowded areas such as shopping malls, can be a frightening experience for people with balance problems. Remember, walking can start a positive cycle which can lead to a more active life-style. Many people with peripheral neuropathy can increase muscle strength and tone to the point where they can utilize other treatment options mentioned in this chapter.

A Proper Shoe and Fit Can Improve Gait and Balance

Choosing the proper shoe for your life style, combined with a proper fit, can greatly improve balance and stability. In order to make a good choice it is important to understand the components of a shoe.

The *toe box* is the tip of the shoe.

The *vamp* is in the center of the shoe near the area where the laces are placed.

The *bottom sole* extends from the bottom of the heel to the toe.

The *insole* is situated inside the shoe and extends from the heel to the toes.

The *heel* is made out of various materials including rubber or synthetic materials and provides elevation of the foot.

The *last* is built into the shoe and determines the curvature of the shoe. Most shoe lasts are made for people with a neutral or normal arch type.

Guidelines for a Proper Fit

- Always have both feet measured and fit the foot with the larger size. If the difference in shoe size varies more than one complete size, you probably need two different size shoes.

- When trying on new shoes wear the type of sock or hose that you intend to normally wear.

- There should be ½-inch space from your longest toe to the end of the shoe.

- Make sure the heel does not slip out of the shoe when you walk.

- A new shoe should be comfortable when you first try it on. Do not anticipate that "you will break in the shoe" as you continue to wear it.

- Since many feet swell as the day progresses, do your shoe shopping in the middle of or at the end of the day.

- It is important that the width of the shoe fits properly. Bulging of the shoe, especially around the great toe, indicates that the shoe is too narrow. Conversely, gapping of the shoes means that the shoe is too wide for your feet.

Lighter Weight Shoes Make Walking Easier

Many people with neuropathy have muscle weakness and unsteadiness. It is much easier to lift the foot when the shoe is constructed out of lightweight leather. Brands that make lightweight shoes include Hush Puppies®, Easy Spirit®, Rockport® and New Balance®. There are many companies that make lightweight shoes. At the Foot Pain Center we suggest that our patients feel the weight of the shoe before trying it on.

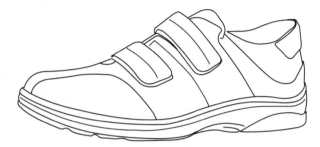

Fig 12: Rocker Bottom Soles Improve Steadiness and Balance

A rocker bottom sole has a more rigid construction and is raised in the toe area. This type of sole creates a "rocking motion," propelling the foot forward from heel to toe, rather than from side to side. The more the toe box is angulated, the greater the correction. Rocker bottom soles are available on many of the better walking shoes such as SAS®, Ecco®, New Balance®, Mephisto® and many others. In some cases, when greater correction is needed to help increase stability, a prescription rocker bottom sole can be added to a shoe.

Arch Supports and Orthotics

Arch supports (also known as foot orthotics) are used to help the foot function normally during the walking cycle. There are three classifications of foot types. The neutral foot has a normal arch structure. The flatfoot has a collapsed and broken down arch. The

high-arch foot has an excessively high in-
step with a greater angulation of the heel
bone. Each foot type requires a different
type of arch support.

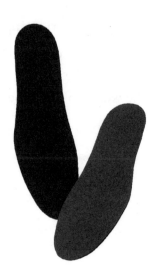

   A neutral foot requires little or no
correction. An arch support or orthotic
may be used to provide extra cushioning
and shock absorption. A runner or power
walker may use an arch support to help
prevent the formation of blisters, calluses
or plantar fasciitis (heel pain).

Spenco

Spenco® is made out of a soft material called neoprene which
offers excellent cushioning.
The Aetrex® brand offers a
number of different types
softer arch supports in different materials and styles.
A person with peripheral
neuropathy who experiences

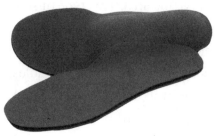

odd sensations—such as the feeling of walking on rocks, marbles
or cardboard—might benefit from this type of support. Power-
Step® innersoles are lightweight, provide shock absorption and fit
into almost any type of shoe.

   Flatfoot deformities have many causes including heredity
factors, injury or the prolonged use of ill-fitting shoes. It is not
uncommon for people with peripheral neuropathy to develop flat-
feet due to diminished muscle strength. Flat feet often require the

use of an orthotic or arch support to support the collapsed arch and also restore normal function during the walking cycle.

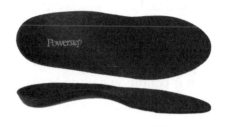

These arches have a build up in the inside arch thus countering the effects of fallen arches.

High-arch feet can be inherited or acquired. Some neurological conditions, such as Charcot-Marie-Tooth disease, can result in a high arch. This condition is one of the many causes of peripheral neuropathy. A person with a high arched foot bears excessive weight on the heel and ball of the foot (metatarsal region). The purpose of an orthotic is to redistribute the weight more evenly throughout the foot. These devices are well-padded in the heel and often have a built-in metatarsal pad to remove pressure from these areas.

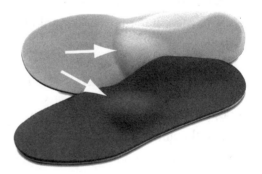

The Use of Braces for Walking and Balance Difficulties

A foot and ankle brace, also known as an AFO (ankle-foot orthosis), can play an important role in treating more serious walking and balance problems. Advances in the field of kinesiology (the science of human motion) have made foot and ankle braces more effective in controlling gait abnormalities and also more cosmetically acceptable. Braces made in earlier decades were cumbersome, heavy and very conspicuous. Today most braces are constructed from lightweight plastics, neoprene and soft leather.

A common condition experienced by peripheral neuropathy sufferers is drop foot deformity. As previously described, drop foot is condition caused by damage to a nerve in the leg called the peroneal nerve. A person with drop foot cannot raise the foot at the ankle during the walking cycle. With the inability to flex or bend the foot at the ankle, a person has to raise the foot and ankle as one unit. This creates a very awkward and highly unstable walking pattern called a high steppage gait. Braces can be very effective in adding much needed stability throughout the gait cycle in drop foot conditions. Generally two types of braces are used for drop foot conditions, articulating and non-articulating braces. Articulating braces have a hinge at the ankle region and assist in raising the foot at the ankle.

Articulating Step-Smart™ Brace

A popular non-articulating brace that does not bend at the ankle, but provides stability for the muscles, tendons and ligaments of the foot and ankle, is called a posterior leaf spring brace.

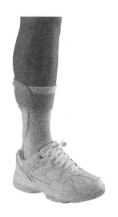

Posterior Leaf Spring Brace

Other neurological conditions where braces are commonly used include Charcot-Marie-Tooth, multiple sclerosis and post-stroke patients.

Chapter 10

Experimental Therapies

Few medical conditions have as many specialty pharmaceutical products in development as pain control. The search for a cure, or at least more effective treatment, for neuropathic pain has become a hot area of research since the publication of "Numb Toes and Aching Soles" in 1999. Drug companies are anxious to access some of the estimated $4 billion peripheral neuropathy market, which is only expected to grow within the next 10 years as the population of North America ages and as diabetes rates continue to escalate. To date, success in the area of pain management has been less than stellar, with very few new pharmaceutical pain medications making it to market in the last 25 years. This chapter will characterize the pipeline of products in development and discuss the implications of these new and novel approaches to the prevention and treatment of neuropathic pain.

Since no one can predict the future, this chapter is at best a survey of promising new treatments. Most neuropathic pain sufferers are interested to know what treatments are available today. However, it is also nice to have a sense that progress is being made on many fronts to improve the treatment options available to neuropathy sufferers. The goals of the research include improved symptom management, finding ways to slow the progress of nerve degeneration, and even therapies to reverse neuropathies altogether.

Having this information now can also help people to understand what strategies scientists are investigating. This understanding can suggest things that neuropathic pain sufferers can do today, such as using nutritional supplements, and even incorporating specific foods into their diet that have a similar mode of action to some of the potential drugs being developed. Every effort will be made to mention practical advice that is relevant. The other purpose for a discussion of experimental therapies is to help people to better handle their present situation with the hope that improved therapies are on the horizon.

One reason that progress in the area of peripheral neuropathy has lagged is the complexity of the condition. As previously discussed, there are many possible causes of peripheral neuropathy. This suggests that there are many ways that nerves can be damaged, just like there are many ways a car can be damaged in an accident. And just as with car accidents, where each accident may require a different corrective measure (i.e. new bumper, new radiator, new engine), scientists are now developing a host of strategies to deal with peripheral neuropathy. In the near future we will see many more options for the treatment of peripheral neuropathy, and many people will likely be using a "cocktail" of medications, much like what is common today for conditions such as HIV, high blood pressure and cancer.

One strategy that researchers are investigating, based on the traditional idea of symptom management such as pain control, involves the development of new types of pain medications. Another strategy involves the development of neuroprotectants. These are substances that have the potential to protect nerves from damage and possibly even allow for some nerve repair. Another approach is to find medications that improve circulation, as many believe that poor blood flow to the nerves is at the root of many cases of peripheral neuropathy. And one of the most promising areas of research is into substance known as "nerve growth factors," which are molecules that can stimulate nerves to grow and repair. Gene therapy and stem cell research, although in the early stages, also have a tremendous potential to lead to a cure for peripheral neuropathy. Let's look at some of these new strategies in more detail.

Neuroprotectants

Preventing Neuropathy in Persons with Diabetes: ARIs and AGEs

The promise of aldose reductase inhibitors (ARIs) and advanced glycation end product (AGE) inhibitors, discussed below, lies in their ability to lessen the severity of neuropathies and increase nerve function in people with diabetes. They do this by overcoming the effects of elevated glucose levels. The hope is that these substances will prevent and even reverse the underlying damage to the nerves in persons with diabetes.

Aldose Reductase Inhibitors (ARIs)

When blood sugars in people with diabetes are above normal levels, the body responds by channeling the excess glucose into other sugar forms such as sorbitol. The conversion of excess glucose to sugar alcohols is known as the "polyol pathway." An accumulation of sorbitol is often found in diabetic nerve tissue where it seems to upset the chemical balance in nerve cells and increase the amount and severity of diabetic neuropathy. The enzyme that converts glucose to sorbitol in the body is called "aldose reductase." The overactivity of this enzyme is thought to cause neurological problems for many people with diabetes. Molecules that reduce aldose reductase activity are called aldose reductase inhibitors (ARIs). The hope is that following their administration for an appropriate period, nerve function will be maintained or restored in people with diabetes and peripheral neuropathy will be mitigated.

**Aldose Reductase Inhibitors:
Synthetic and Naturally Occuring**

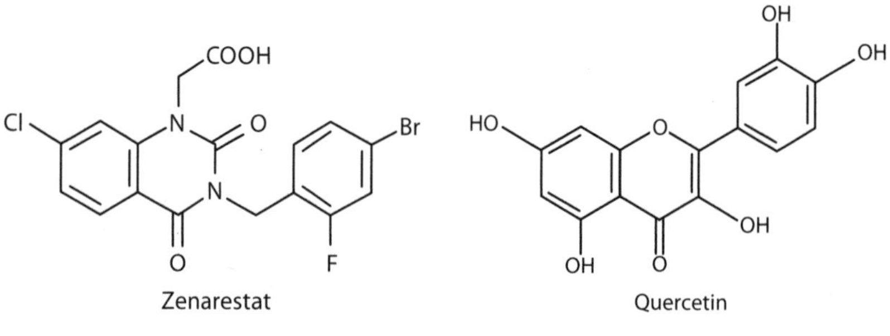

Zenarestat   Quercetin

Fig 13: Aldose Reductase Inhibitors

At this time there are at least three ARIs with promising results in various stages of drug development. Persons with diabetes who took these drugs in clinical trials had improvement in numbness, reduced abnormal sensations, and less cramping and pain. In the same trials the control group (those who were given a placebo) only had a deterioration of their peripheral neuropathy symptoms. Their results were confirmed with electrical testing of nerve conduction. One safety issue that has arisen with these new compounds is potential kidney toxicity, of particular concern to persons with diabetes. Future trials are planned to further assess the safety and efficacy of ARIs.

The AGE and Aminoguanidine Story

Aminoguanidine is a substance that has been known for over 100 years, since it is very similar to guanidine, the active ingredient in the herb goat's rue that has been used as an alternative treatment for diabetes. Just as ARIs inhibit the build-up of sorbitol, aminoguanidine appears to inhibit the development of what are known as "advanced glycation end products" or AGEs. AGEs are simply proteins that have been damaged by sugar, similar to the way the heat of cooking causes "browning" or "caramelization." High levels of AGEs are associated with diabetic peripheral neuropathy. In essence, high sugar levels have "carmelized" the nerve cells in diabetes. Having said that, AGE levels tend to increase with age—even in persons without diabetes. For this reason, aminoguanidine has aroused interest not only for persons with diabetes, but also as an "anti-aging" molecule, since it may be able to prevent some of the signs of aging. By blocking AGE formation, aminoguanidine has shown potential in the reduction of age spot formation and the prevention of cataracts, atherosclerosis, diabetic kidney damage and peripheral neuropathy. Aminoguanidine is available as a nutritional supplement, with a typical dose of 300 mg per day recommended by the literature. A drug based on aminoguanidine called pimagedine is also being developed.

Natural Neuroprotectants

Quercetin, a natural bioflavonoid, has also been shown to be a potent aldose reductase inhibitor. Quercetin is found in many foods, including onions, red wine, tea, apples, berries and brassica family vegetables. As a natural bioflavonoid, quercetin also has been shown to possess anti-inflammatory, antioxidant and cancer prevention properties while having a safe history of use. Quercetin is also available as an orally taken nutritional supplement, with a typical dose being 500 mg three times per day. A topical formulation containing quercetin, called QR-333, is also being developed for peripheral neuropathy with positive clinical results.

There are also many other naturally occurring neuroprotectants found in a wide variety of foods and beverages. Especially of interest to researchers are compounds called polyphenols. These are very potent antioxidants found in dark-pigmented berries (blueberries, strawberries, blackberries), grapes, red wine, green tea, and many other fruits and vegetables. Blueberries, for instance, have been shown to protect animals from a wide range of nerve degeneration-based conditions such as Parkinson's disease and Alzheimer's disease. Based on these findings it makes sense for people with peripheral neuropathy to incorporate foods high in polyphenols into their diet, or take nutritional supplements containing them.

Focus on Blood Flow

It has been suspected for some time that reduced blood flow to nerve cells can promote the development of peripheral neuropathy. If small blood vessels that supply the nerves are not delivering adequate amounts of blood, then the nerve cells are more prone to damage and at the same time less likely to get the nutrients they need to repair. The model for this has been persons with diabetes, who have a tendency to possess compromised circulation. However, compromised blood flow may be a factor in the development of many more cases of peripheral neuropathy. Hence there are a number of approaches that focus on improving blood flow to the nerves to improve the symptoms of peripheral neuropathy.

Protein Kinase Inhibitors

Excess glucose levels tend to increase the production of a substance called diacylglycerol (DAG), which reduces vascular blood flow. Drugs called protein kinase inhibitors are oral medications that prevent DAG formation. They have shown the potential to be an effective therapy for diabetic eye problems (retinopathy), kidney problems (nephropathy), neuropathy, and cardiovascular disease, since all these conditions can result from poor micro-circulation. A number of protein kinase inhibitors are currently under development. Additionally, the antioxidant vitamin E has been identified as an inhibitor of DAG formation, and it shows promise in reducing vascular complications in diabetes. At this time a supplement of natural mixed tocopherol form of vitamin E seems reasonable at a dose of 400 IU per day. Note that the "natural mixed" type of vitamin E is different from the synthetic forms and that it contains all the naturally occurring vitamin E forms. Previous studies of vitamin E have typically used only one form of vitamin E, leading to a relative deficiency of the other forms and less effective results.

Encouraging Blood Vessel Growth and Repair

Vascular endothelial growth factor (VEGF) is another substance receiving a lot of attention from scientists researching peripheral neuropathy. VEGF is a normally occurring substance in the body that stimulates new blood vessel formation. Diabetes, high cholesterol levels and aging cause reduced levels of VEGF. VEGF, administered either through gene therapy or protein injection, is currently under intensive investigation for the potential to prevent and reverse nerve damage. In one experiment, scientists used gene therapy to increase VEGF in rabbits 10 days after nerve function was damaged by lack of blood flow. VEGF-treated rabbits recovered much faster than untreated rabbits. A study of VEGF for the treatment of peripheral neuropathy in humans is currently recruiting patients.

Prostaglandins and Essential Fatty Acids

Prostaglandins are short-acting hormones that affect a variety of cells, such as in blood vessels, causing constriction or dilation. Prostaglandins are also among the most important modulators of inflammation and pain. Since prostaglandins are produced from dietary fats called essential fatty acids, the types of prostaglandins produced can be altered by changing the types of fats consumed in the diet. Saturated fats tend to increase the types of prostaglandins that reduce circulation and increase inflammation and pain. Conversely, omega-3 fats found, for instance, in fish and flax oils tend to improve circulation and reduce inflammation and pain. Therefore, shifting the diet from predominantly saturated (i.e. animal) fats to a diet high in omega-3's can improve circulation and reduce pain. Drugs based on naturally occurring prostaglandins are also in development.

Developments in Pain Control—the Search for the Magic Bullets

The most debilitating symptom for the majority of people with peripheral neuropathy is pain. Many cannot understand how, in this age of the Internet, the supercomputer and the space shuttle, there is no effective treatment for their pain. Or even, for that matter, a way to accurately measure their pain. But pain is very complex, and scientists are only now beginning to understand its intricacies. Pain signals are controlled by a vast and complex communication system that makes New York City air traffic control look like child's play. It has been found that nerves contain a vast array of pain receptors which respond to a wide variety of chemical messages.

One of the first pain medications, morphine, was found to bind to an opioid receptor. Subsequently, it was discovered that morphine does this because it has a chemical structure similar to naturally occurring pain killers called endorphins.

Since that discovery it has been found that there are actually many flavors of pain receptors responding to many different types of chemical messages. This has made it difficult for researchers to isolate the jumbled messages responsible for the pain of peripheral neuropathy. But that is changing, and as a result there are a host of new drugs, noted in Table 2, being developed that bind to some of the most promising receptors believed to be involved in neuropathic pain.

Getting Nerves to Repair

Nerve Growth Factors

Nerve growth factor (NGF) was discovered over 50 years ago as a molecule that promoted the survival and regeneration of neurons. These growth factors are important for the maintenance of neuron health and the regeneration of damaged nerves. Interestingly, it has been shown that there is a reduction of NGF in various diseases, including diabetes. It has also been reported that NGFs increase both the number (three to four fold) and elongation of adult neurons. A number of potential new drugs are being developed based on these findings. It should also be noted that a number of natural substances have shown promise as inducers of NGF production. One of the most interesting is vitamin D3, which is known to be a common nutrient deficiency. Another natural NGF stimulator is the Asian mushroom lion's mane (hericium erinaceus), which was used traditionally by Chinese emperors. Lion's mane has been shown to contain at least two compounds which stimulate NGF, and has shown clinical benefit in Alzheimer's disease patients in Japan.

Gene Therapy

The holy grail for peripheral neuropathy sufferers is the "true cure"—that is, the complete restoration of neurological and physical functions and the consequent disappearance of all symptoms. If and when it is found, it most likely will involve some form of nerve regeneration. One of the most promising ways to induce nerve regeneration is by genetic or gene therapy. This involves supplying DNA material to cells. DNA is essentially a recipe for the manufacture of proteins. By altering the DNA, cells can be programmed to produce new proteins to replace those that may be missing or damaged. Once this takes place the body can keep on making the needed protein as long as those cells live. In effect, the gene becomes the gift that keeps giving.

Currently this treatment is being studied in animals for a number of diseases, including cancer, cardiovascular disease, arthritis, and many types of neurological disorders, including peripheral neuropathy.

In fact, researchers from the University of Pittsburgh School of Medicine successfully used gene therapy to block the pain response in animals with neuropathic pain. They used a genetically-engineered herpes simplex virus (HSV) to deliver the gene for a receptor found primarily on the surface of nerve cells. This gene then manufactured the new receptor (protein) which was incorporated into peripheral nerves. The new receptor, called GlyR, was then stimulated via an injection which effectively turned off the neuropathic pain signal. In another study, gene therapy was used to increase nerve growth factor production in mice, thereby reversing neuropathy in diabetic mice. Although these results with animals are encouraging, human studies are likely five years away and it will likely be at least 10 years before an approved gene therapy treatment is developed.

Stem Cell Technology

The ability of the body to generate entirely new cells to help treat diseases and disorders is another hot area of research. Stem cells are cells that produce all the different types of cells that make up the body, more than 200 cell types in total, including nerve cells. Human stem cells are present in human embryos, aborted fetuses, and to a lesser extent, adults. Since certain types of cells in the body, such as neurons, have less capacity for repair and regeneration, it is easy to see the important therapeutic value of stem cells. Stem cells may be able to overcome this failure by metamorphosing into the kind of cells required, thereby replacing the tissue needed. What is truly exciting is the potential not only for all neurological conditions, including Parkinson's disease and Alzheimer's disease, but also for any degenerative condition of any body tissue. To date, stem cell therapy for neuropathy has been limited to a few cancer patients who also developed neuropathy. In one case, a 40-year-old cabinet maker was given high dose chemotherapy followed by stem cell transplantation. Before treatment he was unable to walk; after treatment his peripheral neuropathy symptoms improved, and 12 months later he was able to walk unaided.

Experimental Topical Approaches

Topical approaches to the treatment of peripheral neuropathy offer some distinct advantages over oral treatments. Since topical medications act locally at the site of application, less is absorbed into the body. The net result is that more of the medicine gets to the place it is needed, and less goes to places where it is not needed. This means there are far fewer chances of side effects or toxicity with topical approaches. The appropriate amount of the drug can be applied as needed, with less concern about systemic effects and strain on organs of detoxification, such as the kidneys and liver. Currently there are at least three promising new topical treatments in development.

NGX-4010

NGX-4010 is a new topical patch based on a synthetic capsaicin known as trans-capsaicin. It has been studied for post-herpetic neuralgia (402 patients) and HIV-associated neuropathy (307 patients) over a 12-week period. The interesting finding from these trials is that a single application of the patch seems to provide up to three months of pain relief. As many people are aware, however, capsaicin products can actually increase pain in the short term, as they work by depleting a pain-promoting compound known as "substance P." In the NGX-4010 studies mentioned, patients were pretreated with another topical local anesthetic, presumably to lessen this effect.

NP-1

NP-1 is a topical cream made up of two existing FDA-approved drugs, the analgesic ketamine and the antidepressant amitriptyline. Both these drugs have shown potential to control neuropathic pain when taken orally; however, at the oral dose necessary to achieve pain control, side effects often limit their use. A Phase II clinical trial of 92 patients with various types of neuropathy showed a response rate for pain control with NP-1 of

46 percent versus 19 percent for placebo. In addition, detectable blood concentrations of the active ingredients were insignificant, and the only side effect noted was skin irritation. Also, the combination of drugs was shown to be more effective than either ketamin or amitriptyline by itself.

QR-333

QR-333 is composed of concentrated and standardized nutrient-based active compounds, dosed in a topical cream. It is designed to reduce oxidative stress and inflammation associated with diabetic peripheral neuropathy. Although the exact method of action for QR-333 is unknown, the antioxidant and anti-inflammatory characteristics of its active compounds have been well established. QR-333 contains quercetin (a flavonoid with aldose reductase inhibitor effects, as mentioned earlier), ascorbyl palmitate (synthetic fat-soluble antioxidant form of vitamin C, which is also known as an aldose reductase inhibitor), and vitamin D3 (which has been shown to induce NGF production). QR-333 was shown in a clinical trial to reduce the severity of numbness and jolting pain in 12 weeks. Improvements were also seen in overall and specific quality-of-life measures. It is likely that QR-333 works more by protecting neurons and encouraging repair than as an analgesic, so longer studies may reveal a continuation of improvement.

Drug Name	Target Receptor	Phase of Development (I-IV)
BVT 115959	Adenosine (A2A)	II
Ralfinamide	Sodium Channels	II
Lacosamide	Sodium Channels	III
NGX-4010	TRPV1	III
Sativex®	Cannabinoid (CB)	III*
Zenvia™	NMDA	III

* Approved in Canada for MS pain

Table 4: Summary of New Drugs in Development

Appendix 1:
Company List and Contact Info

Company Name	Customer Service Line	Website
Aetrix®	201-833-2700	http://www.aetrix.com
Ben-Gay®	1-800-223-0182	http://www.bengay.com
Cymbalta®	1-800-545-5979	http://cymbalta.com
Duloxetine (Cymbalta)®	1-800-545-5979	http://cymbalta.com
Gabapentin (see Neurontin®)	1-800-879-3477	http://www.pfizer.com
Lidoderm®	1-800-462-3636	http://www.lidoderm.com
Lyrica® - DPN and PHN Patients	1-866-459-7422	http://www.lyrica.com
Lyrica®- Fibromyalgia Patients	1-888-559-7422	http://www.lyrica.com
Medi-Rub®	877-Medi-Rub (633-4782)	http://www.medi-rub.com
Neuragen®	1-888-234-7256	http://www.originbiomed.com
Neurontin®	1-800-879-3477	http://www.pfizer.com
Pregabalin (see Lyrica®)	1-866-459-7422	http://www.lyrica.com
Spenco®	1-800-877-3626	http://spenco.com
Taxol®	Contact your Physician	http://www.taxol.com
The Neuropathy Association Inc.®	212-692-0662	http://www.neuropathy.org
Tylenol®	1-877-TYLENOL	http://www.tylenol.com
Zostrix®	866-263-9003	http://www.zostrix.com

Appendix 2:
US Neuropathy Support Groups

ALABAMA
Attn: Mr. Frank Broadway
Central Alabama PN Support
Group
4341 Hillside Oaks Montgomery, AL 36109
Tel: 334-244-2020

ALASKA
N/A

ARIZONA
Mesa / Apache Junction
Ms. Marilyn Falk
Tel: (480) 354-2231
Email: embogey@msn.com
1035 N. Idaho, Apache Junction (Senior Center)

Tucson
Mr. Alex E. McDonald
Tel: (520) 749-3583
Email: debmac100@cox.net
Tucson PN Support Group
Tucson Medical center
5301 E. Grant Road, Tucson, AZ

Scottsdale
Ms. Donna M. Brower
Tel: (480) 312-7984
Email: dbrower@scottsdaleAZ.gov
Civic Center PN Support
Group
Civic Center Senior Center
7375 E. 2nd St., Scottsdale, AZ 85251

ARKANSAS
Mountain Home
Ms. Anita Hayden
Tel: (870) 425-4701
Email: reamh@suddenlink.net

CALIFORNIA
Costa Mesa, California
Marc Spitz, DPM
Tel: (562) 799-0656
Email: footpaincenter@aol.com

The Costa Mesa PN Support
Group
Costa Mesa Senior Center
695 W. 19th Street, 92627
For more information, please
contact Dr. Spitz.

Fullerton, California
Mr. Jack McGouldrick
Tel: 714 256 8273
Email: blcjac@earthlink.net
Morningside Neuropathy Support Gp.
Morningside Commons Saddleback Room
800 Morningside Dr. Fullerton, CA 92835

Los Angeles, California
Mrs. Velda De Cosentine
Email: help@numbtoes.org
Answering Service: 310 485-0357
UCLA Medical Center, Building 300, 3rd Floor Conference Room in Westwood, CA.

Los Osos, California
Mr. Alexander Morrison
Los Osos, California
Day Phone: 805-534-1215
Email Address: amor324@charter.net
Johnson Ave. Church of Christ
Address: 3172 Johnson Ave, San Luis Obispo, CA

Chico, California
Ms. Dorothy Rolls
Tel: 530-899-6944
Ms. Clara Brown
Tel: 530-343-8387
Chico PN Neuropathy Group
Enloe Conference Center
Between 5th and 6th Ave, Esplanade, across form Enloe Medical Center

San Diego, California
Ms. Jean Nurding
E-mail: jnurding@san.rr.com
Clairemont Town Square
Shopping Center
4731 Clairemont Drive, intersection Lakehurst

Northern California Chapter of The Neuropathy Association
Official website:
http://www.pnhelp.org/

ALTURAS
Attn: Box Maxell
530-233-3366

AUBURN
Attn: Bev Anderson
530-389-2416

AUBURN
Charlene Amos
530-885-9865
info@phhelp@org

AUBURN
Bev Anderson
530-389-2416
info@pnhelp.org

BERKELEY
Alan Dampsey
510-527-3568
adampsey@comcast.net

CONCORD
Joe Burbulis
925-930-0300
JOEBCA@AOL.COM

DAVIS
Martha Chandley
916-371-1125
kairoschandley@sbcglobal.net

ELK GROVE
Michael Colozzi
916-421-8103
Artistwin46@yahoo.ca

EUREKA
Audrey Drynan
707-268-8937
muffie2005@suddenlink.net

FOLSOM
Beverly Morford
916-984-4302

FORT BRAGG
Ruth Sparks
707-961-1771
jsparks@msn.org

FRESNO
Maria Chavez
877-437-9787
mariac@fresnoaol.com

GRASS VALLEY
Sally Hearn
530-268-1760
info@pnhelp.org

JACKSON
Darlene Jarnigan
209-296-1760
info@pnhelp.org

LINCOLN
Jim Fulcomer
916-543-9201
jjfulcomer@yahoo.com

LIVERMORE
E. Lorne Stack
925-447-6158
info@pnhelp.org

MERCED
jrsisplus@aol.com
209-383-6269

MODESTO
Mary Hudson
209-526-6439
marlu33@aol.com

MONTEREY
Don & Ann Trout
831-372-6959
935oaks@comcast.net

NAPA
Ron Patrick
707-257-2343
bonjournapa@aol.com

OAKLAND
Kathleen Nagel
510-653-8625
kcnagel@earthlink.net

OAKLAND
Jud Leong
510-538-1327
jsmleong@yahoo.com

PLACERVILLE
Frank Roscoe
530-647-0777
froscoe@comcast.net

REDDING
John Wright
530-337-6570
quailh7@frontiernet.net

RENO
Marsha Campbell
775-851-0499
LadyJane28@sbcglobal.net

ROSEVILLE
Mary Lou Ward
916-485-7723
mary@crward.com

SACRAMENTO
Charles Moore
916-485-7723
chasmoor@surewest.net

SACRAMENTO
Myke Taylor
916-487-2903
Walt_taylor@surewest.net

SACRAMENTO
Anne Fletcher
916-391-3317
anne_fletcher@att.net

SAN FRANCISCO
Amy Mahoney
415-353-2312
Amy.Mahoney@ucsfmedctr.
org

SAN JOSE
Stan Pashote
510-490-4456

SANTA CRUZ
Mary Ann Leer
831-477-1239
maleer@comcast.net

SANTA ROSA
William Quarante
707-544-3238

SONOMA
Joann Bertolucci
707-996-8336

SONORA
L.D.Wright
209-533-2887
klwright30@sbcglobal.net

STOCKTON
Naomi Denby
209-474-3312
theplonusmom@aol.com

SUSANVILLE
Jackie Woodson
530-257-4693
jwoodie@frontiernet.net

TRUCKEE
Jesse Griffin
530-587-5152

WALNUT CREEK
Nancy Ostrander
925-930-9524
onono@pacbell.net

WEST SACRAMENTO
Martha Chandley
916-371-1125
kairoschandley@sbcglobal.net

WOODLAND
Delia Genera
916-661-3238
dgenera@wavecable.com

YREKA
Terry Rees
530-842-1577
tarees@snowcrest.net

YREKA
Gene Arnold
530-842-7744
gene@4fast.net

YUBA CITY
Nancy Escudero
530-673-3698
nancychristina1@yahoo.net

COLORADO
LakeWood
Mr. Jim Williams
Tel: 303 954 9914
Email: jimrwil@comcast.net
Lakewood PN Support Group
Lutheran Church of the
Resurrection
7100 W Mississippi Ave,
Lakewood CO, 80226
The Lakewood PN Group
P. O. Box 19268
Denver, CO 80219

Colorado Springs
Mr. Robert Lowes
Tel: 719-488-5605
Email: bnjlowes@aol.com

View Pointe PN Support
Group
View Point Apartments
555 S. Rockrimmon Road,
Colorado Springs, CO 80909

Denver
Dorothy Miller **President
The Denver Chapter of The
Neuropathy Association
Tel: 303 814-2112
Email: dorothy_miller@
hotmail.com

CONNECTICUT
Roton
Ms. Linda McIntosh
Tel: 860-460-6445
Email: LynMac47@aol.com
Southeastern Connecticut
Neuropathy Support Group,
Waterford, CT at the Waterford
Public Library

DELAWARE
Wilmington
Ms. Frank Castelli
Tel: 302-475-1706
Email: fcastelli@msn.com

D.C.
N/A

FLORIDA
Duval County
Dr. Alan Berger, MD
The Duval Neuropathy Support
Group
Glendale Community Church
6411 Beach Blvd.,
Jacksonville, FL 32216
Tel: 904-244-9922

Broward/Dade Counties
Mr. Eugene Richardson
Tel: 954-523-2987
Email: prcgene@aol.com
The Southeast, FL. Support
Group
North Broward Medical
Center.
201 E. Sample Rd. Pompano
Beach, Fl.

Highland Counties
Mr. Eugene Richarson
Tel: 954-523-2987
Email: prcgene@aol.com

Lee County
Dr. John Lawlar
Tel: 239-573-1001
SW Florida PN Support Group
Lee Memorial Hospital /
Health Park
2776 Cleveland Ave/9918
Health Park Circle
Tel: 239-693-7224

Bradenton
Mr. Neal Kuyper
Tel: 941-761-0179
Email: Neal_Christina@msn.
com

Mr. Joseph Musso, Co-Leader
Tel: 941-753-4283
Palm Beach County

Dr. Samuel Grundfast
Tel: 561-964-0147
Email: grundfa5@aol.com

Mid Palm Beach County PN
Group
JFK Hospital
5301 S. Congress Ave,
Atlantis, FL 33462

PN Support Group
Pinnacle Medical Center
315 75th St. West, Bradenton,
FL 34209

Indian River Counties
Mrs. Lou Nielsen
Mr. Chuck Nielsen, Co-Leader
Tel: 772-287-1292

Ladylake
Ms. Jean Ganske
Tel: 352-753-8382
Email Address: yajyajll@aol.
com
Messages and Announcements:
Lady lake Support Group
North Lake Presbytarian
Church
Rolling Acres Rd, in the
village

Leesburg
Ms. Marion Jansson
Resident Services Coordinator
352.728.8525 ext 507
Email: MJansson@
lakeportsquare.com
The Lake Port Square PN
Group
Lake Port Suqare
800 Lake Port Blvd., Leesburg,
FL 34748

GEORGIA
Metropolitan Atlanta
Mr. James H. Griesmer
Tel: 404-378-3516
Email: griesmerjh@bellsouth.
net

Ms. Hilary Hargreaves, Co-
Leader
Tel: 404-378-4587
Email: hilaryrick@bellsouth.
net

Decatur PN Support Group
Piccadilly Cafeteria
2595 N. Decatur Road,
Decatur GA

HAWAII
N/A

IDAHO
Boise
Ms. Patricia Montross
Tel: 208-395-1547
Email: pmirishman@aol.com

Boise PN Support Group
1994 Wood Duck Lane, Boise,
ID 83706

ILLINOIS
Quad Cities (IL & IA)
Ms. Mary Kay Keemle
Tel: 309-755-1063
Email: mkeemly@sbcglobal.net

East Moline PN Support Group
Illini Hospital, Larson Center,
Suite C, Silvis, IL 61282

Ms. Kathy Slottage
Tel: 773-693-3578
Email: kslottag@aol.com
This is an ON-LINE Group
ONLY. This group does NOT
meet.

INDIANA
Central Indiana
Margaret L. Frazer, M.D.
Tel: 317-844-2903
Email: Margaret.L.Frazer@pfizer.com

Central Indiana Neuropathy
Support Group
St. Lukes Methodist Church
100 W. 86th St., Indianapolis,
Indiana, 46260
Church Tel: 317-846-3404.

IOWA
Doubuque/Tri-State
Mr. Bert Muir
Tel: 563-583-2536
Email: muirsmail@mchsi.com

Cedar Rapids
Ms. Kitty Chandler
Tel: 319-378-8403
Email: Kchand6165@aol.com
Cedar Rapids Peripheral
Neuropathy Support Group
Prairiewoods, 120 E Boyson
Rd, Hiawatha, IA 52233

KANSAS
N/A

KENTUCKY
Bowling Green/Warren City
Mr. Eric McGriff
Tel: 270-783-0805
Email: ejmcgriff@gmail.com

Louisville
Ms. Debbie Goldstein
Tel: 502-426-4399
Email: Dinowriter@insightbb.com

Ms. Peggy Smith, Co-Leader
Tel: 502-239-7239
Email: pegstar@msn.com

Louisville PN Support Group
of Kentuckiana
The Suburban Hospital
4001 Dutchmans Ln,
Louisville, KY

LOUISANA
Baton Rouge
Dr. Richard G. Palecki, D.P.M.
Tel: 225-2910093

Ms. Jennifer Sigler, Co-Leader
Tel: 225-906-4819
Email: jennifer.sigler@nmchbr.
com

Baton Rouge PN Support
Group
NeuroMedical Center, 10101
Park Rowe Avenue
(near corner of Perkins and
Bluebonnet Blvd.)
Baton Rouge, LA 70810, 2nd
floor

MAINE
Bangor Area
Ms. Suzanne Mock
Tel: 207-862-6671
Email: garynsue@msn.com

MARYLAND
Southern Maryland
Mr. David Spore
Tel: 301-737-0623
Email: Dspore@aol.com

Parkville
Ms. Dorothea Svilar
Tel: 410-668-0841

MASSACHUSETTS
North Shore
Mr. Werner Paster
Tel: 978-479-4339
Email: wpaster@comcast.net

North Shore PN Support
Group
Beverly Hospital
Beverly, MA

Lowell Internet Group
Mr. Joseph Moniz
Tel: 508-567-8824
Email: Polyjoee@aol.com

Orleans
Ms. Jackie Stowell
Tel: 508-255-7697
Neuropathy Support Group of
Cape Cod

Orleans Council on Aging
Rock
150 Rock Harbor Rd.,Orleans,
MA. 02653

MICHIGAN
Ms. Dorothy Teesdale
Tel: 616-897-9794
Email: bildot@sbcglobal.net

Mid West Michigan PN
Support Group
St. Paul Anglican Church
2560 Lake Michigan Dr. NW
2nd Wednesday of each Month
(No January & February)

East Michigan Peripheral
Neuropathy Support Group
Mr. Len McCulloch
Tel: 248-474-2763 extension
22
Time: 7:00-8:30pm
Livonia Senior Center
15218 Farmington Road
Livonia 48154

MINNESOTA
Ms. Lois Martin
Phone: 952-941-5372
Email Address: lmemartin@
comcast.net

MISSISSIPPI
N/A

MISSOURI
The St. Louis Chapter of The
Neuropathy Association
President: Kathy Hodgson
Vice President: Scott Hunt
email address for both:
neurop2005@yahoo.com
Contact phone number: 877-
373-7817

Kansas City
Ms. Shirley Lynn
Tel: 913-299-9873
Email: denimladye@yahoo.
com
Meeting Place: St. Lukes Of
Kansas City
Peet Centre, Conference
Room 2, 4401 Wornall Rod.
KC, MO 64111

MONTANA
N/A

NEBRASKA
Ms. Sandy Behrens
Tel: 402-483-4908
Email: lisasmom53@aol.com
Nebraska Neuropathy Support
Group
Bryan LGH Medical Plaza
1600 S. 48th St., Lincoln, NE
68506

Lincoln
Ms. Sandy Behrens
Tel: 402-483-4908
Email: lisasmom53@aol.com

NEVADA
Las Vegas
Ms. Kim Heffner, Leader
Tel: 702-452-8277
Email: KHeffner@levi.com

The Las Vegas Neuropathy
Support Group
The Flamingo Library
Reno, Nevada (Including
Sparks, Spanish Springs, Verdi,
Fernley, Fallon, Carson City,
Incline Village, and Yerington,
NV)

Mrs. Marsha J. Campbell,
Leader
Tel: 775-851-0499 - Cell: 775-
846-3374
Email: LadyJane2B@
SBCglobal.net

**The Reno Neuropathy
Support Group**
Fire Station #11 @ 7105 Mae
Anne Rd. at Sharlands Dr.
(North of I-80 and West of
Robb Drive)

NEW HAMPSHIRE
N/A

NEW JERSEY
W. Essex
Ms. Mary Robertson
Phone: 973-809-4615
Email Address: ithacamom@
comcast.com

Tinton Falls
Ms. Fontainne Gatti
Tel: 908-233-9709
Email: fontainegatti@msn.com
Fontaine.D.Gatti@aexp.com

Rehabilitation Center of Tinton
Falls
2 Centre Plaza
Tinton Falls, NJ 07724
732-460-5320

Englewood
Ms. Mary Robertson/Tom
McCullum
Tel: 973 226 1535/Tel: 201 692
9313
ithacamom@comcast.net/
mcculluma@optonline.net

Northern New Jersey
Peripheral Neuropathy Support
Group:
Meets from 7:30 9:00 p.m. in
Conference Room A/B,
Englewood Hospital in
Englewood, N.J.
Call 201-894-3000 for
directions to the hospital.

Hamilton
Mr. Bill Giovannetti
Tel: 609-587-8039
Email: billpg2000@aol.com

Ms. Frances Burns, Co-Leader
Tel: 609-298-8135
Email: grannyb@snip.net

Robert Wood Johnson PN
Group
Robert Wood Johnson Medical
(Hamilton)
1 Health Hamilton Plaza,
Hamilton, NJ 08690

NEW MEXICO
N/A

NEW YORK
Manhattan
Ms. Irene Beer
Tel: 212-787.2767
Email: IRENESHB@aol.com

Mr. Steven Smith
Tel: 914-310-0490
Email: stevenspuds@
optonline.net

The Manhattan PN Support
Group
Site: CBS building 51 W. 52
St.
(East of 6th Ave. Take elevator
to 33F.)

The West Essex Support Group
The Roseland United
Methodist Church, 144 Eagle
Rock Ave., Roseland, N.J.
Ms. Mary Robertson 973-809-
4615 or ithacamom@comcast.
com

Brooklyn
Ms. Lisa Volpe-Campisi
Tel: 718-232-4179
Email: kellynyc98@aol.com

Herkimer
Ms. Annette K. Reeder
Tel: 315-866-5227
Email: AHR44@juno.com

Rochester
Mr. John McNeill
Tel: 585-247-5543
Email: jmcn1937@frontiernet.
net

PN Support Group of Monroe
County
St. Johns Meadows
(Retirement Community) in
Brighton, Briarwood Club
Room
Mohawk Valley Support Group
Valley Health Center
Contact Annie or Harry at
(315) 866-5227

NORTH CAROLINA
Pittsboro
Ms. Vera Reece
1107 Fearrington Post
Pittsboro, NC 27312
Email: breece@mindspring.
com
Tel: (919) 542-7272
Gathering Place in Fearrington
Village @ Time: 11:00 a.m

Raleigh
Ms. Marion Tice
Tel: 919-872-2360
Raleigh Neuropathy Support
Group
Raleigh Elk Lodge
3558 Millbrook Rd, Raleigh,
NC

Greensboro
Ms. Retta Gray
Tel: 336-852-8489
Email: rgkikinscremin@
bellsouth.net

NORTH DAKOTA
Minot
Mr. Richard Kraft
Tel: 701-776-5127

OHIO
Cleveland/Akron
Ms. Kay Seawright
Tel: 330-468-2526
Email: kjcright@yahoo.com

Greater Cincinnati
Ms. Shirley Planet
Tel: 937-433-1296
Email: planetnews@fuse.net

Greater Cincinnati PN Group
Good Shepard Lutheran
Church
7791 Kenwood Rd, Cincinnati,
OH 45236
Shepard PN Support Group
Shepard Christian Church
9571 Shepard Rd, Macedonia,
OH

Miamisburg
Sandy Daws, LPN
Tel: 937-866-9089
Email: SDaws@
kingstonhealthcare.com

OKLAHOMA
Oklahoma City
Mr. Jim Miller
Tel: 405-605-3649
Email: jmiller238@cox.net

Ms. Janice Coleman
Tel: 405-373-2286
Email: seamanjs@aol.com

Oklahoma City PN Support
Group
Meeting Place: United Life
Church
3332 N. Meridian Meeting

Tulsa
Mary Lou Harkins
Tel: 918-830-0157
Email: cassia1@cox.net
Tulsa PN Support Group
Will Rogers United Methodist
Church
1138 South Yale, Tulsa, Ok.
74112

OREGON
Cornwallis
Ms. Betty McCarty
Tel: 541-926-1212
Email: mccartyjb@comcast.net

Mr. Dave Bethman
Tel: 541-754-9565
Email: dmbethman@comcast.
net

Heart of the Valley PN Support
Group
Corvallis Senior Center
260 NW Tyler Ave, Corvallis,
OR 97330

PENNSYLVANIA
Broomal
Ms. Denise Metz
Tel: 610-356-4719
Email: metz1370@comcast.
net.
Southeastern Pennsylvania
Peripheral Neuropathy Group
Main Line Health Lawrence
PArkCenter Broomall, PA.

Erie
Ms. Louise Schulze
Tel: 814-838-2556
Email: louise230@aol.com
Erie PN Support Group
St. Vincent Health Center - 1st
floor conference room
232 W. 25th Street, Erie, PA

Bryn Mawr
Ms. Donna M. Elberson
Tel: 610-446-0792
Cell: 610-585-9753

Mr. Dean Elberson
Tel: 610-527-3051
Email: nfaaneuropathy@aol.
com

The Never Feel Alone Again
PN Support Group
Place: Bryn Mawr Hospital
Clothier Hall Building, 1st
floor
Lindsay Avenue (Across from
ER)
Bryn Mawr, PA 19010
Bethlehem
Ms. Jasmine Nuesa
Tel: 610-866-6614
Email: jasmin.nuesa@gmail.
com

PUERTO RICO
N/A

RHODE ISLAND
N/A

SOUTH CAROLINA
Columbia
Mr. John Watkins
Tel: 803-256-1957

Ms. Mary Spradlin, Co-Leader
Tel: 803-782-5823
Email: MHSpradlin@aol.com

Columbia Area PN Support
Group
Incarnation Lurtheran Church
at 3005 Devine St

Greenville
Mrs. Patsy Young
Tel: 864-877-0702
Email: patsyy101@aol.com

Palmetton PN Support Group
St Bernidene center
4 St. Francis Dr, Greenville,
SC 29601

Charleston
Richard Marks, M.D.
Tel: 843-884-3573
Email: Bluffhouse@hotmail.
com

Mt. Pleasants PN Support
Groups Group

West Ashley (Group #1)
Meeting Place: St. Joseph
Church
Address: Wallenberg Blvd,
Charleston, SC

East Cooper (Group #2)
Meeting Place: St. Andrews
Church
Address: Wilden St, Mt.
Pleasant, SC

North Area (Group #3)
Meeting Place: Trident
Hospital
Address: Trident Community
Center

SOUTH DAKOTA
Gregory
Ms. Patti Nachtigal, R.N.
Tel: 605-835-8394
Email: Patti.Nachtigal@
gregoryhealthcare.org

Avera Gregory PN Support
Group
Avera Gregory Healthcare
Center
P.O. Box 408, Gregory, SD
57533
Tel: 605-835-8394

TENNESSEE
Memphis
Herbert W. Smith, Ph.D.
Tel: 901-843-3098
Email: hsmith@rhodes.edu

Greater Menphis PN Support
Group
Place: Rhodes College
2000 N. Parkway, Memphis,
TN 38112

Knoxville
Ms. Paula Isenberg
Tel: 865-945-3810
Cell: 865-748-1407
Email: chronicpain@myway.
com

2 Locations:
1) Knoxville meets at Faith
Promise Church (just off
Pellissippi Parkway)
10740 Faith Promise Ln.,
Knox. TN., 37931. Call me or
the church (865-251-2590) for
directions

2) The Powell meeting meets
at 1st Baptist Church of Powell
7706 Ewing Rd., Powell, TN.,
37849. (865-947-9074)

Loudon
Mr. James Fella
Tel: 865-458-1781
Email: tvfella@aol.com

TEXAS
San Antonio
William "Bill" Thomas
Tel: 830-629-5693
Email: wthomas1@satx.rr.com

Corpus Christi
Richard Bates, RN
Tel: 361-992-1464
Cell: 361-945-2255
Email: Rbates825@aol.com

Christi Support Group
South Hospital
Saratoga Blvd., Corpus Christi,
TX

Fort Worth
Mr. Ken Hestand
Tel: 817-737-4735
Email: khestand@charter.net
Name: Ft. Worth Neuropathy

Houston Area
Ms. Ann L. Green
Tel: 281-556-1415
Email: anngreen33@sbcglobal.
net

Houston PN Support Group
Memorial Drive Lutheran
Church
12211 Memorial Drive,
Houston, TX

Arlington
Ms. Mary Heyduck
Tel: 817-496-6298
Email: mapaheyduck@cs.com

Arlington Are PN Support
Group
Place: St. Barnabas United
Methodist Church
5011 W. Pleasant Rd.,
Arlington, TX 76016

Northeast Tarrant County
Mr. James Beard
Tel: 817-318-1639
Email: J.Kbeard@sbcglobal.
net

NE Tarrant County PN Support
Group
SITE: Parc Place Retirement
Facility in Bedford
Rolling Meadows Retirement
Complex

Mr. Joe Castelli
Tel: 940-692-2807
Email: joecastelli5@sbcglobal.
net
Name: The Rolling Meadows
Retirement Complex
For information on this group,
please contact Mr. Joe Castelli
at: (940) 692-2807

UTAH
N/A

VERMONT
N/A

VIRGIN ISLANDS
N/A

WASHINGTON
Bremerton
Ms. Joy Brydon
Tel: 360-479-3626
Email: joybrydon@yahoo.com

The Canterbury Manor PN
Support Group
Canternury Manor
703 Callahan, Bremerton, WA
98310
For more information, please
contact Ms. Joy Brydon at 360-
479-3626

Bellingham
Mr. William M. Ouwennel
Tel: 360-676-0367
Email: billouw@comcast.net

Northwest PN Support Group
St. Lukes Community Health
Education Ctr
3333 Squalicum Parkway,
Bellingham, WA

VIRGINIA
Virgina Beach
Mr. Robert M. Williamson
Tel: 757-518-8086
Email: williamson23@aol.com

Tidewater Neuropathy Support
Group
Meeting Place: Private Dining
Room, Sentara Bayside
Hospital
Address: 800 Independence
Blvd, Virginia Beach, VA
Meeting Schedule: 2nd
Saturday of each month
(except July,. Aug., and Dec.)

Fairfax County
Ms. Iris Sax
Tel: 703-548-9062
Neuronova PN Support Group
George Mason Government
Center
Fairfax, VA

WEST VIRGINIA
N/A

WISCONSIN
Northeast/Fox Valley
Mr. Michael Barklow
Tel: 920-380-0218
Email: mb40@att.net

Mr. Ron Fafnis, Co-Leader
Tel: 920-687-9196
Email: rfafnis@sbcglobal.net

N.E.W PN Support Group
Our Savior Lutheran Church
3009 N. Meade Street,
Appleton, WI 54911

The Positive Thinkers PN
Support Group
Ms. Mary Yellick
Tel: 800-272-3666

Ms. Carolyn Meitler
Tel: 262-968-4631
Email: cmeitler@wi.rr.com

Positive Thinkers PN Support
Group
Froedert Medical
9200 W, Wisconsin Rd,
Milwaukee, WI Meeting

WYOMING

Casper

Ms. Doris Hlava
Tel: 307-234-1976
Email: DorisQMD@AOL.Com
Casper PN Support Group
Central Wyoming Senior
Center
1831 East 4th St, Casper, WI
82601

Appendix 3:
Neuropathic Pain Questionnaire

Neuropathic Pain Questionnaire
Please answer Yes or No to each Question

Can your pain be described as;

Hot, as in feels like the area is "burning"	Yes ❏ No ❏
Cold, as in feels like the area is "freezing"	Yes ❏ No ❏
Sharp, as in feels like a "knife wound"	Yes ❏ No ❏
Shooting, as in feels like an "electric shock"	Yes ❏ No ❏
Prickling, as if on "pins and needles"	Yes ❏ No ❏

Do you experience any other sensations in the same area as the pain, such as:

Tingling, as if "ants are crawling over your skin"	Yes ❏ No ❏
Itchiness, like a "mosquito bite"	Yes ❏ No ❏
Numbness, as in "lack of sensation"	Yes ❏ No ❏

Is the pain sometimes worse from light touch such as clothing?   Yes ❏   No ❏

Do you have muscle weakness, "heaviness", cramping, or temperature variation in the same area as the pain.   Yes ❏   No ❏

Yes = 1 Point, No = 0 Points

Total out of a possible 10 points: _____

If total is equal or greater than 4, it is very likely that you have neuropathic pain.

Index

vitamin (continued)

  E 16, 51, 53-55, 63-64, 68,
      70, 73-76, 80-83, 92,
      149, 152-155, 169, 195-
      196, 198, 202

vomiting 110-112, 169

W

walking difficulty 8

weakness 8, 10-11, 13, 18-20,
  23, 30, 32, 103, 176, 178,
  180-181, 184

weight gain 65, 104, 113, 130

World Health Organization
  (WHO) 36, 167

WTSmed.com 169

Z

Zostrix® 134

BOOK ORDER FORM

(Order extra copies for any friends or relatives you think might benefit – even for your doctor!)

Telephone orders: Call 1-888-MED-9898 toll free (1-888-633-9898)

Online orders: Go to medpress.com

Fax orders: Fax the form you have filled in below to 1-902-492-0013

Postal orders: Mail the form you have filled in below to:

> *MedPress, PO Box 81, Halifax,*
> *Nova Scotia, Canada B3J 2L4*

Please send me the following:

> *Nutrients for Neuropathy*
>
> _____ copies (paperback), $22.95 each
>
> *Numb Toes and Aching Soles: Coping with Peripheral Neuropathy*
>
> _____ copies (paperback), $24.95 each
>
> _____ copies (professional case bound edition), $29.95 each
>
> *Numb Toes and Other Woes: More on Peripheral Neuropathy*
>
> _____ copies (paperback), $24.95 each
>
> _____ copies (professional case bound edition), $29.95 each

Shipping & Handling

> Please add for U.S. deliveries, $7 for first book, $3 for each additional book. For shipments outside the U.S., please call 1-888-633-9898 or email orders@medpress.com for information.

Payment: _____ Check (payable to "MedPress")

> _____ Credit Card:
> The undersigned hereby consents to payment for orders
> to be charged to a credit card listed below:

Authorised Signature: _____

Print Name on Card: _____

Exp Date: _____

Credit Card Number: _____

Card Type: Visa ____ Mastercard ____ AMEX ____

3-Digit Code (req'd): _____

Corresponding Address for Credit Card: _____

_____

Corresponding Telephone Number for Credit Card: _____